Critical

Care

Notes

Clinical Pocket Guide

Janice Jones, PHD, RN, CNS
Brenda Fix, MS, RN, NP

Purchase additional copies of this book at
your health science bookstore or directly from
F. A. Davis by shopping online at www.fadavis.com
or by calling 800-323-3555 (US) or 800-665-1148
(CAN)

A Davis's Notes Book

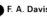 F. A. Davis Company · Philadelphia

F. A. Davis Company
1915 Arch Street
Philadelphia, PA 19103
www.fadavis.com

Printed in China by Imago

Last digit indicates print number: 10 9 8 7 6 5 4 3 2 1

Director of Content Development: Darlene D. Pedersen
Acquisitions Editor: Jonathan Joyce
Senior Developmental Editor: William F. Welsh
Project Editor: Meghan K. Ziegler

Reviewers:
Lisa Ann Behrend, RN, MSNc, CCRN-CSC
Deborah Little, MSN, RN, CCRN, CNRN, APRN, BC
Janice Garrison Lanham, RN, MSN, CCNS, FNP

Danette Wood, EdD, MSN, RN, CCRN
Laura Carousel, MSN, RN, CCRN
Jeanie Krause-Bachand, MSN, EdD, RN, BC
Deborah Pool, MS, RN, CCRN

As new scientific information becomes available through basic and clinical research, recommended treatments and drug therapies undergo changes. The author(s) and publisher have done everything possible to make this book accurate, up to date, and in accord with accepted standards at the time of publication. The author(s), editors, and publisher are not responsible for errors or omissions or for consequences from application of the book, and make no warranty, expressed or implied, in regard to the contents of the book. Any practice described in this book should be applied by the reader in accordance with professional standards of care used in regard to the unique circumstances that may apply in each situation. The reader is advised always to check product information (package inserts) for changes and new information regarding dose and contraindications before administering any drug. Caution is especially urged when using new or infrequently ordered drugs.

Sticky Notes

✓HIPAA Compliant
✓OSHA Compliant

**Waterproof and Reusable
Wipe-Free Pages**

Write directly onto any page of *Critical Care Notes*
with a ballpoint pen. Wipe old entries off
with an alcohol pad and reuse.

BASICS	CV	RESP	GU	NEURO	GI	HEMA/ONCO	ENDO
MULTISYS	CC MEDS	TOOLS					

Look for our other Davis's Notes Titles

*For a complete list of Davis's Notes and other titles for health
care providers, visit www.fadavis.com.*

Physical Assessment

Reusable Assessment Form

Name:	Room:	Age:
Diagnosis:		
Surgeries/Past Hx:		
Activity:	Diet:	DNR/DNI:
Allergies:		
Neurological/MS: ICP:		

Cardiac:
  VS/A-line:
  ECG:
  Hemodynamics: PAD   PAS   PCWP   CVP
  IABP:		

Respiratory:
  Ventilator:
  ABGs/SpO$_2$:		

GI:		
GU:		
Wounds/Incisions:		
Drainage Tubes:		
Treatments:		
Special Needs:		
Other:		

Normal Arterial and Venous Blood Gases

Blood Gas Components	Arterial	Venous
pH	7.35–7.45	7.31–7.41
PO_2	80–100 mm Hg	35–40 mm Hg
PCO_2	35–45 mm Hg	41–51 mm Hg
HCO_3	22–26 mEq/L or mmol/L	22–26 mEq/L or mmol/L
Base Excess (BE)	–2 to +2 mEq/L or mmol/L	–2 to +2 mEq/L or mmol/L
O_2 saturation	95%–100%	68%–77%

Blood Gas Results

Arterial		Venous
	pH	
	PO_2	
	PCO_2	
	HCO_3	
	Base Excess (BE)	
	O_2 saturation	

Quick Blood Gas Interpretation

Acid-Base Disorder	pH	PCO_2	↑ HCO_3
Respiratory acidosis	↓	↑	↑ if compensating
Respiratory alkalosis	↑	↓	↓ If compensating
Metabolic acidosis	↓	↓ if compensating	↓
Metabolic alkalosis	↑	↑ if compensating	↑

Full or total compensation: pH will be within normal limits

Compensation:

- Respiratory problem → the kidneys compensate by conserving or excreting HCO_3^-
- Metabolic problem → the lungs compensate by retaining or blowing off CO_2

Also look for mixed respiratory and metabolic problems.

$PaCO_2$ or HCO_3^- in a direction opposite its predicted direction or not close to predictive value.

Common Causes of Acid-Base Imbalances

Respiratory acidosis	COPD, asthma, head injury, pulmonary edema, aspiration, pneumonia, ARDS, pneumothorax, cardiac arrest, respiratory depression, CNS depression, or head injury
Respiratory alkalosis	Hyperventilation, anxiety, fear, pain, fever, sepsis, brain tumor, mechanical overventilation
Metabolic acidosis	Diabetes mellitus, acute and chronic renal failure, severe diarrhea, alcoholism, starvation, salicylate overdose, pancreatic fistulas
Metabolic alkalosis	Loss of gastric acid (vomiting, gastric suction), long-term diuretic therapy (thiazides, furosemide), excessive $NaHCO_3$ administration, hypercalcemia

Pulse Oximetry

SpO_2 monitoring: Monitoring saturation of peripheral O_2

SpO_2 Level	Indication
>95%	Normal
91%–94%	May be acceptable, provide O_2 as necessary, encourage C&DB or suction prn
85%–90%	Provide O_2 as necessary, encourage C&DB or suction prn, may be normal for COPD patient
<85%	Prepare for possible intubation

False readings may occur because of anemia, CO poisoning, hypothermia, hypovolemia, peripheral vasoconstriction caused by disease or medications.

Lactic Acidosis

Lactic acid is a byproduct of anaerobic metabolism. Increased levels indicate inadequate perfusion of vital organs with resultant tissue hypoxia. May result from inadequate perfusion and oxygenation of vital organs; post cardiac or respiratory arrest; cardiogenic, ischemic, or septic shock; drug overdoses, seizures, cancers, or diabetes mellitus.
Critical values: Blood pH, <7.35, and lactate >5–6 mEq/L or >45 mg/dL.
Treat with sodium bicarbonate IV if acidosis is readily evident.

Capnography

Capnography is the measurement, display, and monitoring of the concentration or partial pressure of CO_2 ($PETCO_2$) in the respiratory gases at the end of expiration. The capnogram displays the maximum inspiratory and expiratory CO_2 concentrations during a respiratory cycle, which indirectly reflect the production of CO_2 by the tissues and the transport of CO_2 to the lungs. Sudden changes in CO_2 elimination should be monitored in selected cardiorespiratory patients and postoperatively after major cardiothoracic surgeries. Capnography can also be used to verify ETT position and monitor the effectiveness of CPR.

Causes of ↑ PᴇᴛCO₂	Causes of ↓ PᴇᴛCO₂
Fever	Hypothermia
Hypertension	Hypotension
Increased cardiac output	Decreased cardiac output
Hypoventilation	Hyperventilation
Hypovolemia	Hypervolemia
Airway obstruction	Airway obstruction
Bronchial intubation	Accidental extubation
	Pulmonary embolus
	Cardiac arrest
	Apnea

Normal range of ᴇᴛCO₂ is 35–45 mm Hg

↑ RR (hyperventilation) → ↓ CO₂ → ᴇᴛCO₂ < 35 = respiratory alkalosis

↓ RR (hypoventilation) → ↑ CO₂ → ᴇᴛCO₂ > 45 = respiratory acidosis

There are five characteristics of the capnogram that should be evaluated: frequency, rhythm, height, baseline, and shape.

Normal Capnogram

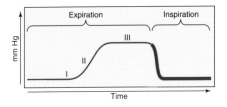

Phases I, II, and III represent expiration, the bolded lines represent inspiration. Long periods of a flat wave form indicate apnea, dislodged endotracheal tube, esophageal intubation, or patient disconnect from ventilator.

BASICS

Artifical Airways and Mechanical Ventilation

Artifical Airways

Endotracheal Tube
- Adult oral tube sizes: Males 8.0–8.5, I.D. (mm); females 7.0–8.0. I.D. (mm) (internal diameter).
- Placement is 2 cm above the carina. Verify by auscultating for breath sounds bilaterally, uniform up-and-down chest movement, CXR, and checking end-tidal CO_2 immediately after intubation.
- Cuff pressure: 20–25 mm Hg.

Tracheostomy Tube
- Size will vary.
- Cuff pressure: 20–25 mm Hg.

Minimal leak technique or minimal occluding volume verifies that an ETT or tracheostomy tube is at its lowest inflation point. Attach a 10-mL syringe to the balloon of the inflated cuff. Position your stethoscope on the patient's neck at the area of the carotid pulse. Inflate balloon cuff to a point where no leak is heard. Slowly remove air from the inflated cuff until you hear a slight leak at the height of inspiration. Then add 1 mL of air back into the cuff.

Cuff pressure can also be monitored via a calibrated aneroid manometer device. Connect manometer to cuff. Deflate cuff. Reinflate cuff in 0.5 mL increments until desired cuff pressure is achieved. Check cuff pressure every 8–12 hrs or per agency protocol.

Mechanical Ventilation

Classification of Ventilators
Positive Pressure Ventilation

- **Volume-Cycled Ventilator:** Delivers a preset constant volume of air and preset O_2.
- **Pressure-Cycled Ventilator:** Produces a flow of gas that inflates the lung until the preset airway pressure is reached.
- **Time-Cycled Ventilator:** Programmed to deliver a volume of gas over a specific time period through adjustments in inspiratory-to-expiratory ratio.

■ **High-Frequency Jet Ventilator (HFJV):** Delivers 60–100 bpm with low tidal volumes under considerable pressures.

Negative Pressure Ventilation

Uses the old iron lung principle by exerting a negative pressure on the chest wall to cause inspiration. No intubation required. Custom fitted "cuirass" or "turtle" shell unit that fits over the chest wall. May be utilized at night for patients who require assistance during sleep.

Modes of Ventilation

■ **Controlled Mechanical Ventilation (CMV):** Machine controls rate of breathing. Delivery of preset volume (TV) and rate regardless of patient's breathing pattern. Sedation or paralyzing agent (e.g., Pavulon) usually required.

■ **Assist Controlled Ventilation (ACV):** Patient controls rate of breathing. Inspiratory effort triggers delivery of preset volume.

■ **Intermittent Mandatory Ventilation (IMV):** Patient breathes spontaneously (own tidal volume) between ventilator breaths of a preset volume and rate.

■ **Synchronized Intermittent Mandatory Ventilation (SIMV):** A form of pressure support ventilation. Administers mandatory ventilator breath at a preset level of positive airway pressure. Monitors negative inspiratory effort and augments patient's spontaneous tidal volume or inspiratory effort. Synchronized with patient's breathing pattern.

■ **Positive End-Expiratory Pressure (PEEP):** Increases oxygenation by increasing functional residual capacity (FRC). Keeps alveoli inflated after inspiration. Can use lower O_2 concentrations with PEEP; decreases risk of O_2 toxicity. Ordered as 5–10 cm H_2O.

■ **Continuous Positive Airway Pressure (CPAP):** Maintains positive pressure throughout the respiratory cycle of a spontaneously breathing patient. Increases the amount of air remaining in the lungs at the end of expiration. Less complications than PEEP. Ordered as 5–10 cm H_2O.

■ **Bilevel Positive Airway Pressure (BiPAP):** Same as CPAP but settings can be adjusted for both inspiration and expiration.

■ **Pressure Support Ventilation (PSV):** Patient's inspiratory effort is assisted by the ventilator to a certain level of pressure. Patient initiates all breaths and controls flow rate and tidal volume. Decreases work of breathing.

- **Inverse Ratio Ventilation (IRV):** All breaths are pressure limited and time cycled. Inspiratory time usually set longer than expiratory time.

IMV, SIMV, CPAP, BiPAP and PSV can all be used in the weaning process.

Weaning
Sample Criteria for Weaning: Readiness
- Alert and cooperative
- $FIO_2 \leq$ 40%–50% and PEEP $\leq$ 5–8 cm H_2O
- Hemodynamically stable
- pH $\geq$ 7.34
- PaO_2 >80 mm Hg
- $PaCO_2$ <45 mm Hg
- PaO_2/FIO_2 ratio >200
- Vital capacity 15 mL/kg and minute ventilation <10
- Hemoglobin >7–9 g/dL and serum electrolytes within normal limits
- Spontaneous respirations >6 b/min. or <35 b/min.
- Negative inspiratory pressure –30 cm H_2O
- Relatively afebrile with limited respiratory secretions
- Inotropes reduced or unchanged within previous 24 hrs
- Sedation discontinued

Weaning Methods
- **T-tube weaning:** Place patient on T-tube circuit on same FIO_2 as on ventilatory assistance. Monitor ABGs after 30 min. Provide a brief rest period on the ventilator as needed and continue to monitor ABGs until satisfactory. Extubate when patient is rested, good spontaneous respiratory effort, and ABGs within acceptable parameters.
- **IMV/SIMV weaning:** Decrease IMV rate every 1–4 hrs. Monitor spontaneous breaths. Obtain ABGs within 30 min. of ventilator change. Allows for gradual change from positive-pressure ventilation to spontaneous-pressure ventilation.
- **PSV:** Use low levels of PSV (5–10 cm H_2O). Decrease in 3–6 cm of H_2O increments. Useful in retraining respiratory muscles due to long-term ventilation.

■ **CPAP/BiPAP:** Provides expiratory support, maintains positive intrathoracic pressure. BiPAP adds inspiratory support to CPAP. Prevents respiratory muscle fatigue.

Nursing assessment during weaning
■ Vital signs and hemodynamics (PAS, PAD, PCWP, CO, CI)
■ Dysrhythmias or ECG changes
■ Oxygenation/Efficiency of gas exchange
■ CO_2 production and elimination
■ pH level
■ Bedside pulmonary function tests
■ Work of breathing including use of accessory muscles
■ Level of fatigue
■ Patient discomfort
■ Adequate nutrition

Ventilator Alarms

Ventilator alarms should never be ignored or turned off. They may be muted or silenced temporarily until problem is resolved.

Checklist of Common Causes of Ventilator Alarms
Patient causes:
■ Biting down on endotracheal tube
■ Patient needs suctioning
■ Coughing
■ Gagging on endotracheal tube
■ Patient "bucking" or not synchronous with the ventilator
■ Patient attempting to talk
■ Patient experiences period of apnea

Mechanical causes:
■ Kinking of ventilator tubing
■ Endotracheal tube cuff may need more air
■ Leak in endotracheal tube cuff
■ Excess water in ventilator tubing
■ Leak or disconnect in the system
■ Air leak from chest tube if present
■ Malfunctioning of oxygen system
■ Loss of power to ventilator

Pathophysiological causes:
- Increased lung noncompliance, such as in ARDS
- Increased airway resistance, such as in bronchospasm
- Pulmonary edema
- Pneumothorax or hemothorax

Nursing Interventions
- Check ventilator disconnects and tubing.
- Assess breath sounds, suction as needed.
- Remove excess water from ventilator tubing.
- Check endotracheal cuff pressure.
- Insert bite block or oral airway.

If cause of the alarm cannot be found immediately or cause cannot be readily resolved, remove patient from ventilator and manually ventilate patient using a resuscitation bag.

Call respiratory therapy stat.

Continue to assess patient's respiratory status until mechanical ventilation is resumed.

Ventilator Complications	
Complication	**Signs & Symptoms/Interventions**
Barotrauma or volutrauma—acute lung injury, may result in pneumothorax or tension pneumothorax, pneumomediastinum, pneumoperitoneum, subcutaneous crepitus	• High peak inspiratory and mean airway pressures • Diminished breath sounds • Tracheal shift • Subcutaneous crepitus • Hypoxemia Insert chest tube or needle thoracostomy.
Intubation of right mainstem bronchus	• Absent or diminished breath sounds in left lung • Unilateral chest excursion Reposition ETT.

Continued

Ventilator Complications—*Cont'd*

Complication	Signs & Symptoms/Interventions
Endotracheal tube out of position or unplanned extubation	• Absent or diminished breath sounds Note location of tube at the lip (21–22 cm). Reposition ETT or reintubate. Restrain only when necessary.
Tracheal damage due to excessive cuff pressure (>30 cm H_2O)	• Blood in sputum when suctioning • Frequent ventilator alarm Monitor ETT cuff pressure every 4–8 hrs. Perform minimal leak technique. Ensure minimal occluding volume.
Damage to oral or nasal mucosa	• Skin breakdown or necrosis to lips, nares, or oral mucous membranes Reposition tube side-side of mouth every day. Apply petroleum jelly to nares. Provide oral care with toothbrush every 2 hrs.
Aspiration Tracheo-esophageal fistulas	• Feeding viewed when suctioning • If blue dye is used, sputum is blue in color Use blue dye with enteral feedings if aspiration suspected. Keep head of bed 30–45 degrees. Administer proton pump inhibitors or histamine H_2-receptor antagonists.
Ventilator-assisted pneumonia Respiratory infection Increased risk of sinusitis	• Refer to section on VAP Assess color and odor of sputum. Monitor temperature, WBC count, ESR.
Decreased venous return → decreased cardiac output due to increased intrathoracic pressure	• Hypotension • Decreased CVP, RAP, and preload Monitor vital signs and hemodynamics.

Continued

Continued

Ventilator Complications—Cont'd

Complication	Signs & Symptoms/Interventions
Stress ulcer and GI bleeding	• Blood in nasogastric drainage • Hematemesis and/or melena Hematest nasogastric drainage, emesis, feces. Administer proton pump inhibitors or histamine H_2-receptor antagonists.
Paralytic ileus	• Absence of diminished bowel sounds Provide nasogastric drainage with intermittent suction. Turn and position patient frequently.
Inadequate nutrition, loss of protein	• Refer to section on nutrition. Start enteral feedings if appropriate. Start total parenteral nutrition if GI tract nonfunctional or contraindicated.
Increased intracranial pressure	• Changes in level of consciousness • Unable to follow commands Assess neurological status frequently.
Fluid retention due to increased humidification from ventilator, increased pressure to baroreceptors causing a release of ADH	Assess for edema. Administer diuretics. Drain ventilator tubing frequently.
Immobility	Turn and position patient frequently.
Skin breakdown	Assess skin for breakdown. Assist patient out of bed to chair unless contraindicated. Keep skin clean and dry, sheets wrinkle-free.
Communication difficulties	Keep communication simple. Obtain slate or writing board. Use letter/picture chart. Communicate using sign language.

Ventilator Complications—*Cont'd*

Complication	Signs & Symptoms/Interventions
Urinary tract infection	• Urine becomes cloudy, concentrated, odorous Change/remove Foley catheter. Ensure adequate hydration. Administer antiinfectives.
Deep vein thrombosis	• Painful, swollen leg; pain may increase on dorsiflexion Assess for pulmonary embolism. See respiratory section. Administer heparin or enoxaparin.
Psychosocial concerns: fear, loss, powerlessness, pain, anxiety, sleep disturbances, nightmares, loneliness	• Anxious • Difficulty sleeping • Poor pain control Administer anxiolytics, sedatives, analgesics. Cluster activities to promote periods of sleep. Allow patient to make choices when appropriate. Allow for frequent family visits. Keep patient and family informed.

Hemodynamic Monitoring

Hemodynamic Parameters

Arteriovenous oxygen difference . . . . 3.5–5.5 vol% or 4–8 L/min
Aortic pressure:

- Systolic . . . . .100-140 mm Hg
- Diastolic . . . . .60–80 mm Hg
- Mean . . . . .70–90 mm Hg

Cardiac output (CO = HR X SV) . . . . .4–8 L/min
Cardiac index (CO/BSA) . . . . .2.5–4 L/min
Central venous pressure (CVP) . . . . .2–8 mm Hg
** Same as right atrial pressure (RAP)
Cerebral perfusion pressure (CPP) . . . . .2–6 mm Hg or 5–12 cm H_2O
Coronary artery perfusion pressure (CAPP) . . . . .60–80 mm Hg
Ejection fraction (Ej Fx or EF) 60%–75%
Left arterial mean pressure . . . . .4–12 mm Hg
Left ventricular systolic pressure . . . . .100–140 mm Hg
Left ventricular diastolic pressure .0–5 mm Hg
Left ventricular stroke work index (LSWI) . . . . .30–50 g/beats/m^2
Mean arterial pressure (MAP) . . . . .70–100 mm Hg
Oxygen consumption (VO$_2$) . . . . .200–250 mL/min
Oxygen delivery (Do$_2$) . . . . .900–1100 mL/min
Pulmonary artery pressure (PAP):

- Systolic . . . . .20–30 mm Hg
- Diastolic . . . . .10–20 mm Hg
- Mean . . . . .10–15 mm Hg

Pulmonary capillary wedge pressure (PCWP) . . . . .4–12 mm Hg
Right arterial mean pressure . . . . .2–6 mm Hg
Right ventricular pressure:

- Systolic . . . . .20–30 mm Hg
- Diastolic . . . . .0–8 mm Hg
- End Diastolic . . . . .2–6 mm Hg

Right ventricular stroke work index (RSWI) . . . . . . .7–12 g/m^2/beat
Pulmonary vascular resistance (PVR) . . . . .20–130 dynes/sec/cm^{-5}
Pulmonary vascular resistance index (PVRI) . . . . . . .200–400 dynes/sec/
cm^5/m^2
Pulmonary ventricular stroke index . . . . .5–10 g/beat/m^2
Right atrial pressure (RAP) . . . . .2–6 mm Hg
Stroke index (SI) . . . . .30–650 mL/beat/m^2
Stroke volume (SV = CO/HR) . . . . .60–100 mL/beat
Systemic vascular resistance (SVR) . . . . .900–1,600 dynes/sec/cm^{-5}
Systemic vascular resistance index . . . . . .1,360–2,200 dynes/sec/cm^{-5}/m^2
Systemic venous oxygen saturation (SvO$_2$) 60%–80%

Cardiac Output Components

Preload	Contractility	Afterload
PaO_2	SaO_2	Hemoglobin (Hgb)
Right atrial pressure	Stroke volume	Pulmonary vascular resistance
Central venous pressure	Cardiac output	Systemic vascular resistance
Left ventricular end diastolic pressure	Tissue perfusion	Blood pressure

Pulmonary Artery Catheter

The purpose of the pulmonary artery catheter, also known as the Swan-Ganz catheter, is to assess and monitor left ventricular function and can determine preload, assess contractility, and approximate afterload.

PCWP approximates left atrial pressure and left ventricular end diastolic pressure.

Increases in PCWP, LAP, or LVEDP indicates heart failure, hypervolemia, shock, mitral valve insufficiency, or stenosis. Decreases in PCWP, LAP, or LVEDP indicate hypovolemia.

PA Catheter Waveforms

The pulmonary artery catheter is threaded through the right atrium and right ventricle and into the pulmonary artery. Insertion is done via fluoroscopy or monitoring waveform changes.

Catheter advanced to right atrium, balloon is inflated. Pressure is low, usually 2–5 mm Hg.	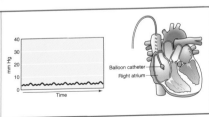

Catheter is floated to right ventricle with the balloon inflated. Waveforms indicate a systolic pressure of 25–30 mm Hg and a diastolic pressure of 0–5 mm Hg.

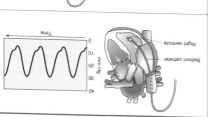

As the catheter moves into the pulmonary artery, the systolic pressure remains the same but the diastolic pressure elevates to 10–15 mm Hg.

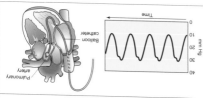

The catheter is moved until it can be wedged in a smaller vessel. When the balloon is inflated, the pressure recorded is that pressure in front of the catheter. It is an approximate measure of the left ventricular end diastolic pressure.

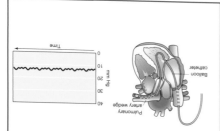

Problems with Pulmonary Artery Catheters

Problem	Check For/Action
No waveform	• Loose connections • Tubing kinked or compressed • Air in transducer • Loose/cracked transducer • Stopcock mispositioned • Occlusion by clot: Aspirate as per policy
Overdamping (smaller waveform with slow rise, diminished or absent dicrotic notch)	• Air bubble or clot in the system • Catheter position: Reposition patient or have patient cough • Kinks or knotting • Clot: Aspirate as per policy
Catheter whip (erratic waveform, variable and inaccurate pressure)	• Catheter position: Reposition patient or catheter; obtain chest x-ray
Inability to wedge catheter (no wedge waveform after inflating balloon)	• Balloon rupture: Turn patient on left side; check catheter position for retrograde slippage

Complications of Pulmonary Artery Catheters

- Risk for infection
- Altered skin integrity
- Air embolism
- Pulmonary thromboembolism
- Cardiac tamponade
- Dysrhythmias
- Altered cardiopulmonary tissue perfusion due to thrombus formation; catheter in wedged position leading to pulmonary infarction
- Catheter displacement/dislodgement
- Loss of balloon integrity or balloon rupture
- Pneumothorax
- Hemothorax

- Frank hemorrhage
- Pulmonary artery extravasation
- Pulmonary artery rupture

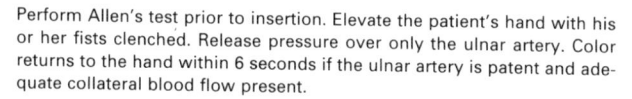

Intra-Arterial Monitoring

An arterial line (A-line) is used if frequent blood pressure and arterial blood gas determinations are needed. It is especially useful

- After surgery.
- For patients with unstable vital signs.
- For patients experiencing hypoxemia.

Perform Allen's test prior to insertion. Elevate the patient's hand with his or her fists clenched. Release pressure over only the ulnar artery. Color returns to the hand within 6 seconds if the ulnar artery is patent and adequate collateral blood flow present.

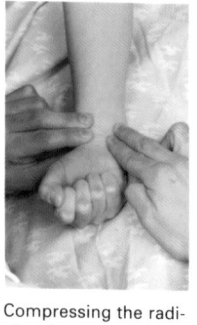

Compressing the radial and ulnar arteries

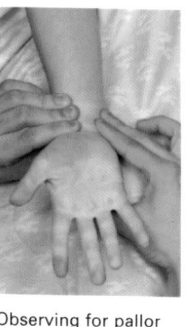

Observing for pallor

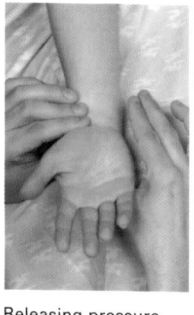

Releasing pressure and observing for return of normal color

Intra-Arterial Waveform

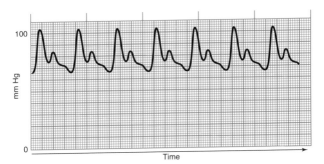

Components of Waveform

- **Systolic peak:** Ventricular ejection and stroke volume. Sharp rise and rounded top.
- **Dicrotic notch:** Aortic valve closure, end ventricular systole, start ventricular diastole. Should be one-third or greater of height of systolic peak. If lower → suspect ↓ C.O.

Tapering of down stroke following dicrotic notch

Important assessments: changes in capillary refill/blanching, sensation, motion, or color that may indicate lack of perfusion to the extremity

$$\text{MAP} = \frac{\text{systolic BP} + (\text{diastolic BP} \times 2)}{3} = 70\text{–}100 \text{ mm Hg}$$

Decreased tissue perfusion—decreasing urine output, elevation in BUN:Creatinine ratio, altered mental status with decreasing level of consciousness, restlessness, dyspnea, cyanosis, dysrhythmias, abnormal ABGs, weak or absent peripheral pulses, increased capillary refill time (>3 sec), diminished arterial pulsations, bruits.

Potential Complications of Intra-Arterial Monitoring

- Hemorrhage
- Air emboli
- Equipment malfunction/inaccurate pressure
- Dysrhythmias
- Infection
- Altered skin integrity
- Impaired circulation to extremities

Nutrition Issues in Critical Care

Primary Concerns

- Starvation and catabolism
- Stress hypermetabolism
- Fluid volume deficit
- Fluid volume excess

Stress and Nutrition

Prolonged or continual stress depletes glycogen stores → hypermetabolic state.

Metabolic rate increases with the release of catecholamines + glucagon + cortisol → hyperglycemia and "stress diabetes."

Protein is lost via gluconeogenesis → decrease in serum protein (albumin).

Lipolysis → increase in free fatty acids.

Nitrogen excretion increases.

Body weight decreases.

1 kg body weight = 1 liter of fluid retained or lost.

Body Mass Index

BMI is a simple means of classifying sedentary (physically inactive) individuals of average body composition and may indicate obesity. It is calculated by the following: Body mass index (BMI) = weight (kg) ÷ height (meters)^2

$$1 \text{ kg} = 2.2 \text{ lbs} \qquad \text{Normal BMI} = 20\text{--}25 \text{ kg/m}^2$$

A BMI >30 kg/m^2 indicates obesity, >40 kg/m^2 indicates morbid obesity. An increase in BMI has been associated with heart disease and diabetes.

A BMI <18.5 kg/m^2 suggests a person is underweight. A BMI <17.5 may indicate the person has anorexia or a related disorder.

BMI does not take into account factors such as frame size and muscularity.

Signs and Symptoms of Fluid Volume Deficit: Hypovolemia

- Dry mucous membranes; dry cracked tongue
- Thirst
- Poor skin turgor
- Sunken eyeballs
- Subnormal temperature
- Decreased or orthostatic blood pressure
- Weak, rapid heart rate and increased respiratory rate
- Decreased capillary refill
- Urine output decreased (<30 mL/hr)
- Increased specific gravity of urine (<1.030)
- Decreased central venous pressure
- Increased hemoglobin and hematocrit
- Increased BUN and serum osmolarity
- Increased BUN:creatinine ratio
- Lethargy, mental confusion

Signs and Symptoms of Fluid Volume Excess: Hypervolemia

- Crackles in lungs; dyspnea, shortness of breath
- Decreased hemoglobin and hematocrit
- Decreased specific gravity of urine
- Distended neck veins and jugular venous pressure
- Edema and decreased serum osmolarity
- Full, bounding pulse; tachycardia
- Increased BP, CVP, and PAP

- Mental confusion, restlessness
- Moist mucous membranes
- Pulmonary congestion or pleural effusion
- Weight gain

Enteral Tube Feedings

Gastric Access
- Nasogastric tube (NGT)
- Oral
- Percutaneous endoscopic gastrostomy (PEG)
- Nasoduodenal tube (NDT)
- Low-profile gastrostomy device (LPGD)

Small Bowel Access
- Nasal-jejunal tube (NJT)
- Percutaneous endoscopic jejunostomy (PEJ)

Types of Tube Feedings

- **Intermittent or bolus feedings**: A set volume of formula is delivered at specified times.
- **Continuous feedings**: A set rate of formula is delivered over a period of time.
- **Cyclic feedings**: Similar to a continuous feeding but the infusion is stopped for a specified time within a 24-hour period, usually 6–10 hours.

Checking Tube Placement

- Aspirate gastric contents and check pH.
  - Gastric aspirate pH 1–4 but may be as high as 6 if patient is on medication to reduce gastric acid (famotidine, ranitidine, pantoprazole).
  - Small intestine aspirate pH $\geq$6.
- Obtain chest x-ray.
- Inject 20–30 mL of air into the tube while auscultating over the epigastrium. Air in the stomach can be heard via a swooshing sound.

Tube-Feeding Formulas

Standard	Very High-Protein/Wound-Healing
Pediatric	Fiber-Containing
Diabetic	Elemental and Semi-Elemental
Pulmonary	Immune-Enhancing or Stress Formulas
Renal	Concentrated

Feeding Tube Complications

Mechanical Complications	Interventions
Nasopharyngeal discomfort	• Reposition tube.
Esophageal ulceration or bleeding esophageal varices	• Consider PEG or PEJ tube.
Clogged tube	• Flush with lukewarm water after every feeding. Hosp. Protocol:
Tube displacement	• Reposition tube.
Extubation	• Insert new tube. • Consider PEG or PEJ tube.
Stomal leak or infection	• Keep area around stoma clean and dry.
Nonmechanical Complications	**Interventions**
Nausea, vomiting, cramps, bloating, abdominal distention	• Withhold or decrease amount, rate, and frequency of feedings. • Change to low-fat formula.
Diarrhea	• Withhold or decrease amount, rate, and frequency of feedings.
Aspiration	• Hold feedings. Check residuals. • Keep HOB elevated 30°–45° during feedings and 1 hr. after bolus feedings.

Continued

Feeding Tube Complications—Cont'd

Nonmechanical Complications	Interventions
Gastric reflux	• Hold feedings. Check residuals. • Keep HOB elevated 30°–45°.
Dumping syndrome: nausea, vomiting, diarrhea, cramps, pallor, sweating, ↑ HR	• Withhold or decrease amount, rate, and frequency of feedings.

Checking for Residuals

1. Assess every 4–6 hrs for continuous feeding and prior to bolus feeding.
2. Using a 30- to 60-mL syringe, withdraw gastric contents from the feeding tube. Note volume of formula.

Volume	Indication
<50 mL	Normal residual.
50-100 mL	Repeat measurement of residual every 1–2 hrs.
>100 mL	Stop feeding. Check residual after 3–4 hrs. When residual is <100 mL, resume feeding at slower rate, amount, or frequency.

Total Parenteral Nutrition (TPN)

TPN is an IV solution of 10%–50% dextrose in water (CHO), amino acids (protein), electrolytes, and additives (vitamins, minerals, trace elements of insulin, vitamin K, zinc, famotidine). Fat emulsions provide fatty acids and calories. Solutions >10% dextrose must be infused via a central line.

■ 1000 mL 5% D/W with 50 g sugar = <200 calories
■ 1000 mL 25% dextrose contains 250 g sugar = 1000 calories

Indications
■ Severe malnutrition
■ Burns

24

- Bowel disorders (inflammatory disorders, total bowel obstruction, short bowel syndrome)
- Severe acute pancreatitis
- Acute renal failure
- Hepatic failure
- Metastatic cancer
- Postoperative major surgery if NPO >5 days

Nursing Care

- Each bag of TPN should be changed at least every 24 hrs with tubing change.
- Monitor intake and output and weigh the patient daily.
- Monitor glucose levels, including finger stick blood sugars every 4 to 6 hours. Cover with regular insulin as necessary. If poor control of serum glucose, consider adding insulin to TPN and continue rainbow coverage.
- Monitor serum electrolytes including magnesium, phosphate, triglycerides, prealbumin, CBC, PT/PTT, and urine urea nitrogen.
- Assess IV site for redness, swelling, and drainage.
- Change gauze dressing around IV site every 48 to 72 hours, as per protocol. Transparent dressings may be changed every 7 days.
- If TPN is temporarily unavailable, hang 10% D/W at the same rate as TPN. Monitor for hypoglycemia.
- Place TPN on infusion pump. Monitor hourly rate. Never attempt to "catch up" if infusion not accurate.
- Patients generally are taken off of TPN prior to surgery.

Complications

Complications from TPN may be catheter-related, mechanical, or metabolic.

Complications of TPN	Signs and Symptoms
Infection, catheter-related sepsis, septicemia, septic shock	Leukocytosis; fever; glucose intolerance; catheter site red, swollen, tender; drainage
Hypoglycemia Blood glucose <70 mg/dL	Shaking, tachycardia, sweating, anxious, dizziness, hunger, impaired vision, weakness, fatigue, headache, irritability

Continued

Complications of TPN	Signs and Symptoms
Hyperglycemia Blood glucose >200 mg/dL	Extreme thirst, frequent urination, dry skin, hunger, blurred vision, drowsiness, nausea
Prerenal azotemia	↓ BUN and serum Na⁺, signs of dehydration, signs of lethargy, coma
Hepatic dysfunction	↓ serum liver function tests (SGOT, SGPT, alkaline phosphatase)
Pneumothorax, hydrothorax Subclavian/carotid artery puncture	SOB, restlessness, dyspnea, signs of hypoxia, chest pain radiating to back, arterial blood in syringe, tachycardia, pulsatile blood flow, bleeding from catheter site
Air embolus	Respiratory distress, dyspnea, SOB, tachycardia, ↑ BP, neurological deficits, cardiac arrest
Dysrhythmias	Atrial, junctional, and ventricular arrhythmias; ↑ C.O., ↓ BP, loss of consciousness
Hypo-/hypernatremia	Normal values: 135–145 mEq/L or 135–145 mmol/L
Hypo-/hyperkalemia	Normal values: 3.5–5.0 mEq/L or 3.5–5.0 mmol/L
Hypo-/hyperphosphatemia	Normal values: 3.0–4.5 mg/100 mL or 1.0–1.5 mmol/L
Hypo-/hypermagnesemia	Normal values: 1.5–2.0 mEq/L or 0.8–1.3 mmol/L
Hypo-/hypercalcemia	Normal values: 8.5–10.5 mg/100 mL or 2.1–2.6 mmol/L

Infectious Diseases

Critical Care Risk Factors

- Invasive devices
- Immunocompromising conditions
- Serious underlying illness
- Prolonged stay in critical care unit
- Colonization and cross-infection

- Overuse of antibiotics
- Elderly

Methicillin-Resistant *Staphylococcus aureus* (MRSA)

Etiology
Health-care associated bloodstream and catheter-related infections. Transmitted by close contact with infected person. Health-care worker may be colonized with MRSA strain with absence of symptoms. The *Staph. aureus* bacterium is resistant to methicillin, amoxicillin, penicillin, oxacillin, and other antibiotics.

Signs and Symptoms
- **Skin infection:** Boil or abscess
- **Surgical wound:** Swollen, red, painful, exudate (pus)
- **Bloodstream:** Fever, chills
- **Lung infection/pneumonia:** Shortness of breath, fever, chills
- **Urinary tract:** Cloudy urine, strong odor

Diagnosis
- Culture of infected area

Treatment
- Vancomycin (Vanocin, Vancoled)
- Linezolid (Zyvox)
- Daptomycin (Cubicin)

Clostridium Difficile (C-diff)

Etiology
C. difficile is a common cause of antibiotic-associated diarrhea (AAD) and is transmitted through the feces or any surface, device, or material that has become contaminated with feces.

Signs and Symptoms
- Watery diarrhea (at least 3 BMs/day for 2 or more days)
- Fever
- Loss of appetite
- Nausea
- Abdominal pain and tenderness

Diagnosis
- Stool culture

Treatment
- Discontinue antibiotics. May give metronidazole (Flagyl) to treat diarrhea

Revised CDC Guidelines 2007

- Perform hand hygiene after touching blood, body fluids, secretions, excretions, and contaminated items immediately after removing gloves and between patient contacts.
- Alcohol-based hand gels are the preferred method for hand decontamination between patients. Decontamination should be performed after contact with a patient and/or medical equipment.
- Gloves and gown should be worn when in contact with clothing or exposed skin with blood or body fluids, secretions, and excretions.
- Mask, eye protection (goggles), and face shield should be worn during procedures such as suctioning or endotracheal intubation if splashes or sprays of body fluids or blood may occur. For patients with suspected or proven infections transmitted by respiratory aerosols, such as SARS, a fit-tested N95 or higher respirator should also be worn.
- For injected medications, single-dose vials are preferred to multiple-dose vials.

During patient transport, masks are not necessary if the patient is wearing a mask. Health-care workers should continue to wear masks when caring for patients with droplet precautions. For more information: http://www.cdc.gov/ncidod/dhqp/pdf/guidelines/Isolation2007. pdf

Psychosocial Issues in Critical Care

Sensory Overload and Deprivation

- **Sensory Overload:** A condition in which sensory stimuli are received at a rate and intensity beyond the level that the patient can accommodate.
- **Sensory Deprivation:** A condition in which the patient experiences a lack of variety and/or intensity of sensory stimuli.

Types of Sensory Stimuli

- Visual
- Auditory
- Kinesthetic
- Gustatory
- Tactile
- Olfactory

Signs and Symptoms of Sensory Problems

- Confusion
- Hallucinations
- Lethargy
- Behavioral changes (combativeness)
- Increased startle response
- Disorientation
- Anxiety
- Restlessness
- Panic
- Withdrawal
- Mood swings
- Withdrawal

Near-Death Experience

The experience of patients that they have glimpsed the afterlife when coming close to death. These perceptions may include:

- Seeing an intense light
- Seeing angels or departed loved ones
- Traveling through a tunnel

Out-of-Body Experience

The experience of being away from and overlooking one's body. The patient feels that the mind has separated from the body.

Family Needs of the Critical Care Patient

- Relief of anxiety.
- Assurance of competent care.
- Timely access to the patient.
- Accurate and timely information about the patient's condition and prognosis in easily understandable terms.
- Early notification of changes in the patient's condition.
- Explanations regarding the environment, machinery, and monitoring equipment.
- Honest answers to questions.
- Emotional support.
- Regard for the spiritual needs of the family and patient.

Organ Donation

Transplantable organs include:
- Kidneys
- Heart
- Lungs
- Liver
- Pancreas
- Intestines

Corneas, the middle ear, skin, heart valves, bone, veins, cartilage, tendons, and ligaments can be stored in tissue banks and used to restore sight, cover burns, repair hearts, replace veins, and mend damaged connective tissue and cartilage in recipients.

Healthy adults between the ages of 18 and 60 can donate blood stem cells: marrow, peripheral blood stem cells, and cored blood stem cells.

Nursing Role in Organ Donation
- Provide accurate information regarding donation.
- Identify possible donors early.

- Work closely with the organ procurement organization and members of the health team to illicit donations.
- Provide emotional support to families considering donation, making sure to respect their cultural and religious beliefs.
- Become a donor advocate among colleagues and for patients and their families.

General Criteria for Brain Death

- Absence of purposive movement
- Flaccid tone and absence of spontaneous or induced movements
- Persistent deep coma
- Absence of spontaneous respiration
- Absence of brainstem reflexes:
  - Midposition or pupils fixed and dilated
  - No corneal, gag, or cough reflexes
  - Absence of spontaneous oculocephalic (doll's eye phenomenon) reflex
  - No vestibular response to caloric stimulation
- Isoelectric or flat electroencephalogram (EEG)
- Absent cerebral blood flow

These criteria vary from state to state.

Hemodynamic management of potential brain-dead organ donors: ensure adequate intravascular volume and adequate cardiac output to ensure consistent perfusion to vital organs.

- MAP $\geq$60 mm Hg
- Urine output $\geq$1.0 mL/kg/hr
- Left ventricular ejection fraction $\geq$45%

Nursing care
- Fluid management—fluids or diuretics
- Inotropic agents to correct low cardiac output
- Vasopressors to correct vasodilatation
- Thyroid hormone
- Corticosteroids to reduce inflammation
- Vasopressin to support renal function
- Insulin to control glucose levels

- Regulate ventilator settings including use of PEEP
- Suction frequently to promote adequate oxygenation

Specific organ donation protocols:

_____
_____
_____
_____
_____
_____
_____
_____
_____
_____
_____
_____

Sedation, Agitation, and Delirium Management

Purpose of sedation is to minimize use of neuromuscular paralysis agents. This will ↓ ventilatory time, ↓ length of stay in ICU, ↓ costs, fewer tracheostomies, and provide early intervention of neurological deterioration. Sedatives should be titrated without impairing neurological assessment. Analgesics should be titrated to keep pain level <3 on 0–10 scale.

Assessment

Prior to sedation, exclude and treat possible causes of agitation and confusion:

- Cerebral hypoperfusion
- Cardiac ischemia
- Hypotension
- Hypoxemia or hypercarbia (elevated blood CO_2)
- Fluid and electrolyte imbalance: acidosis, hyponatremia, hypoglycemia, hypercalcemia, hepatic or renal insufficiency
- Infection
- Drug-induced

Use nonpharmacologic therapies such as massage, distraction, minimize noise. Cluster activities to allow for uninterrupted periods of sleep. Assess pain on 0–10 scale or faces scale and look for nonverbal cues.

Medications for Sedation, Pain, and Delirium

Benzodiazepines
- Diazepam (Valium)
- Lorazepam (Ativan)
- Midazolam (Versed)

Keep antidote flumazenil (Romazicon) available.

Narcotics
- Morphine sulfate
- Codeine
- Fentanyl
- Hydromorphone (Dilaudid)
- Oxycodone (OxyContin)
- Remifentanil (Ultiva)

Alpha-adrenergic Receptor Agonists
- Clonidine (Catapres)
- Dexmedetomidine (Precedex)

Neuroleptics/Antipsychotics/Butyrophenones
- Haloperidol (Haldol)
- Droperidol (Inapsine)

Sedatives/Hypnotics
- Propofol (Diprivan)

Physiological Responses to Pain and Anxiety

- Tachycardia
- Diaphoresis
- Sleep disturbance
- Hypertension
- Tachypnea
- Nausea

Signs of Sedative or Analgesic Withdrawal
- Nausea, vomiting, diarrhea
- Cramps, muscle aches
- Increased sensitivity to pain

- Tachypnea, ↑ HR, ↑ BP
- Delirium, tremors, seizures, agitation

Medication Management

- Monitor body and limb movements, facial expression, posturing, muscle tension for signs of pain.
- Monitor for acute changes or fluctuations in mental status, LOC, disorientation, hallucinations, delusions.
- Evaluate arousability.
- Monitor neurological status including pupillary response, response to verbal commands and pain.
- Monitor respiratory rate and respiratory effort, respiratory depression, BP, HR.

Sedation Assessment Scales

Sedation-Agitation Scale (SAS)

Score	Level of Sedation-Agitation	Response
7	Dangerous agitation	Pulling at endotracheal tube, thrashing, climbing over bed rails
6	Very agitated	Does not calm, requires restraints, bites endotracheal tube
5	Agitated	Attempts to sit up but calms to verbal instructions
4	Calm and cooperative	Obeys commands
3	Sedated	Difficult to rouse, obeys simple commands
2	Very sedated	Rouses to stimuli; does not obey commands
1	Unarousable	Minimal or no response to noxious stimuli

Reprinted with permission from Riker, R. et al. Critical Care Medicine, 1994, 22(3), 433-440.

Bispectral Index Monitoring (BSI)

Physiological assessment of sedation: Examines the EEG and monitors states of increased and diminished cortical arousal. Scoring:

0	Isoelectric brain activity (flat EEG)
40–60	General anesthesia
60–70	Deep sedation
70–80	Moderate (conscious) sedation
90–100	Awake state

Pain Visual Analog Scale (VAS)

no pain 0 _____ worst pain 10
no anxiety   5   severe anxiety

Delirium Assessment

Delirium has been associated with poor patient outcomes. Patients with delirium have higher ICU and hospital stays along with a higher risk of death.

It is characterized by an acute onset of mental status changes that develop over a short period of time, usually hours to days. It may fluctuate over the course of a day. It may be combined with inattention and disorganized thinking or altered level of consciousness. The DSM IV describes three clinical subtypes: hyperactive, hypoactive, and mixed. Hyperactive delirium may be confused with anxiety and agitation.

Benzodiazepines may cause or worsen delirium.

Haloperidol (Haldol) is the drug of choice to treat delirium in the ICU patient.

The Confusion Assessment Method for the Intensive Care Unit (CAM-ICU) score has been used to screen for delirium in the ICU population.

Complications of Sedation, Agitation, and Delirium Therapy

- Hypotension
- Patient unresponsiveness
- Respiratory depression
- Delayed weaning from mechanical ventilator
- Complications associated with immobility: pressure ulcers, thromboembolism, gastric ileus, hospital-acquired pneumonia

Acute Coronary Syndrome (ACS)

ACS is the term used to denote any one of three clinical manifestations of coronary artery disease:

- Unstable angina
- Non-ST elevation MI
- ST elevation MI

Pathophysiology

Unstable angina represents the progression of stable coronary artery disease to unstable disease. Rupture of atherosclerotic plaque causes thrombus formation and partial occlusion in coronary arteries.

Clinical Presentation

ACS presents with chest pain, diaphoresis, SOB, nausea and vomiting, dyspnea, weakness, and fatigue. Look for symptoms of MI—midsternal chest pain, may be described as pressure, squeezing, fullness, or pain. May radiate to jaw, neck, arms, or back and usually lasts more than 15 minutes.

Assessment for chest pain and associated symptoms of ACS include: Use of PQRST method when assessing pain, physical exam, vital signs, auscultate for S3 or S4 gallop, auscultate lungs for crackles, and assess peripheral vessels for pulse deficits or bruits.

Diagnostic Tests

- ECG
- Echocardiogram
- Cycle cardiac markers (troponin I, CK, CK MB, myoglobin, C-reactive protein)

Management

- Administer oxygen to maintain SaO$_2$ >90%.
- Establish IV access.

- Perform cardiac monitoring.
- Administer SL nitroglycerin tablets or oral spray, every 5 minutes x 3 doses. If pain persists, IV nitroglycerin may be started.
- Monitor for hypotension and headaches from vasodilatation.
- Administer aspirin and have patient chew it, if not already on daily dose.
- Administer IV morphine, 2–4 mg every 15 minutes until pain is controlled.
- Monitor for hypotension and respiratory depression.
- Unless contraindicated, administer a beta blocker.

Unstable Angina

Unstable angina is the sudden onset of chest pain, pressure, or tightness due to insufficient blood flow through coronary arteries.

Pathophysiology

Atherosclerosis → obstruction of coronary arteries → decrease blood flow through coronary arteries → decrease oxygen supply to myocardial demand for O_2 during exertion or emotional stress → angina.

Clinical Presentation

Chest pain presents as substernal pain, tightness, dullness, fullness, heaviness or pressure, dyspnea, syncope, pain radiating to arms, epigastrium, shoulder, neck, or jaw.

Women may experience more atypical symptoms such as back pain; GI symptoms, such as indigestion, nausea and vomiting, and abdominal fullness; whereas men may experience typical symptoms such as midsternal chest pain radiating into the left arm.

Diagnostic Tests

- 12-lead ECG
- Lab work: cardiac markers: creatine kinase (CK), creatine kinase-myocardial band (CK-MB), troponin I (TnI), and myoglobin
- Exercise or pharmacological stress test

- Echocardiogram.
- Nuclear scan
- Cardiac catheterization and coronary artery angiography

Management

- Bedrest.
- Obtain ECG and lab work.
- Assess chest pain for frequency, duration, cause that triggered pain, radiation of pain, and intensity based on pain scale from 1 to 10, with 1 being no pain and 10 being worst pain.
- Supply O_2.
- Pharmacological treatment:
    - Early conservative, for low-risk patient: Anti-ischemic, antiplatelet, and antithrombotic drug therapy; stress and treadmill tests.
    - Early invasive: Same drug therapy as early conservative but followed by diagnostic catheterization and revascularization.
    - Administer nitroglycerin (NTG): 0.4 mg (SL or spray) → IV infusion start @ 10 mcg/hr, titrate for pain; check for contraindications such as hypotension, or if taking the following meds: Viagra, Cialis, or Levitra.
    - Administer morphine sulfate IV if symptoms persist after receiving NTG or in patients who have pulmonary congestion or severe agitation.
    - Administer beta blocker: metoprolol.
    - Administer ACE inhibitors in patients with LV dysfunction or CHF with HTN, not recommended in patients with renal failure.
    - Administer calcium channel blockers: Verapamil (Calan, Isoptin) or diltiazem (Cardizem) if patient not responding from beta blocker or nitrates.

Use severe caution when combining blocking agents

    - Administer antiplatelet: Aspirin 160–325 mg, chewed.
    - Administer GP IIb- IIIa inhibitor: Eptifibatide (Integrilin) or tirofiban (Aggrastat) if no contraindications (i.e., bleeding, stroke in past month, severe HTN, renal dialysis, major surgery within the past 6 weeks, or platelet count <100,000 mm^3).
    - Administer antithrombotic: Heparin.
    - Administer anticoagulant: Enoxaparin (Lovenox).

Acute Myocardial Infarction (AMI)

AMI is the acute death of myocardial cells due to lack of oxygenated blood flow in the coronary arteries. It is also known as a heart attack.

Pathophysiology

Injury to the artery's endothelium → increases platelet adhesion → inflammatory response causing monocytes and T lymphocytes to migrate in the intima → macrophages and smooth muscle distend with lipids, forming fatty streaks and forming fibrous cap → thinning of cap increases susceptibility to rupture or hemorrhage → rupture triggers thrombus formation and vasoconstriction → result: thrombus with narrowing artery. If occlusion lasts more than 20 minutes it leads to AMI.

Clinical Presentation

AMI presents with chest pain or discomfort lasting 20 minutes or longer. Pain can be described as pressure, tightness, heaviness, burning, or a squeezing or crushing sensation, located typically in the central chest or epigastrium; it may radiate to the arms, shoulders, neck, jaw, or back.

Discomfort may be accompanied by weakness, dyspnea, diaphoresis, or anxiety, not relieved by NTG. Women may experience atypical discomfort, SOB, or fatigue. Diabetic patients may not display classic signs & symptoms of AMI. Elderly may experience SOB, pulmonary edema, dizziness, altered mental status.

ST-segment elevation MI: Look for tall positive T waves and ST-segment elevation of 1 mm or more above baseline.

Non-ST segment elevation MI: May include ST-segment depression and T-wave inversion.

Diagnostic Tests

- ECG findings
- Cardiac markers (CK, myoglobin, and troponins)

Management

- Focus on pain radiation, SOB, and diaphoresis.
- Obtain a 12-lead ECG and lab draw for cardiac markers.
- MONA: morphine, O_2, NTG, and 160–325 mg aspirin, po. If allergic to aspirin, give ticlopidine (Ticlid) or clopidogrel (Plavix).
- Administer supplemental O_2 to maintain SpO_2 >90%.
- Administer SL NTG tablets or spray.
- Administer IV morphine 2–4 mg every 15 minutes until pain is controlled. (Monitor for hypotension and respiratory depression.)

Hypertensive Crisis

Hypertensive crisis is defined as a severe elevation in blood pressure (systolic BP >179 mm Hg, diastolic BP >109 mm Hg), which may or may not lead to organ damage. There are two types of hypertensive crisis:

- **Hypertensive emergency:** Rapid (hours to days) marked elevation in BP → acute organ tissue damage.
- **Hypertensive urgency:** Slow (days to weeks) elevation in BP that usually does not lead to organ tissue damage.

Pathophysiology

Any disorder or cause (essential hypertension, renal parenchymal disease, renovascular disease, pregnancy, endocrine drugs, autonomic hyper-reactivity, CNS disorder) → ↑ BP → vessel becomes inflamed → leak fluid or blood to the brain → CVA → long-term disability.

Clinical Presentation

Hypertensive crisis presents with

- Chest pain
- Dyspnea
- Neurological deficits
- Occipital headache
- Visual disturbance
- Vomiting

Diagnostic Tests

- CT scan of chest, abdomen, and brain
- 2-D echocardiogram or transesophageal echocardiogram
- ECG
- Lab draws: CBC, cardiac markers, BUN, creatinine, UA, urine toxicology

Management

- Administer O_2 to maintain PaO_2 >92%.
- Obtain VS-orthostatic BP every 5 min, then longer intervals.
- First-line medical therapy: Labetalol (Trandate) and adrenergic-receptor blocker with both selective alpha-adrenergic and nonselective beta-adrenergic receptor blocking actions.
- Administer vasodilator: Nitroprusside (Nipride) and NTG.
- Hypertensive emergency: IV route is preferred; reduce mean arterial pressure (MAP) by no more than 25% in the first hour; if stable, ↓ diastolic BP to 100–110 mm Hg over the next 2–6 hours.
- If pt has neurological complication, primary goal → maintain adequate cerebral perfusion, control HTN, minimize cerebral edema; ↓ BP by 10% but no more than 20%–30% from initial reading.
- Hypertensive urgency: PO meds; ↓ BP in 24–36 hours; short-acting agents: captopril (Capoten) or clonidine (Catapres).

Congestive Heart Failure (CHF)

CHF, which is sometimes referred to as "pump failure," is a general term for the inadequacy of the heart to pump blood throughout the body. This deficit causes insufficient perfusion to body tissues with vital nutrients and oxygen.

Pathophysiology

There are two types of CHF failure: Left-sided failure and right-sided failure. Both may be acute or chronic and mild to severe, caused by HTN, CAD, or valvular disease, involving the mitral or aortic valve. CHF can also be divided into two subtypes: systolic heart function and diastolic heart function.

- Systolic heart function results when the heart is unable to contract forcefully enough, during systole, to eject adequate amounts of blood into the circulation. Preload increases with decreased contractility and afterload increases as a result of increased peripheral resistance.
- Diastolic heart failure occurs when the left ventricle is unable to relax adequately during diastole. Inadequate relaxation prevents the ventricle from filling with sufficient blood to ensure adequate cardiac output.

Clinical Presentation

Left-sided CHF presents as:

- Dyspnea
- Diaphoresis
- Orthopnea
- Tachycardia
- Tachypnea
- Paroxysmal nocturnal dyspnea
- Fatigue
- Pulmonary crackles
- Wheezes
- S3 gallop
- Frothy pink-tinged sputum
- Weakness
- Confusion
- Restlessness

Right-sided CHF presents as:

- Right upper quadrant pain
- Peripheral edema
- JVD
- Hepatomegaly
- Hepatojugular reflux and edema
- HTN
- Anorexia
- Nausea

Diagnostic Tests

- B-type natriuretic peptide (BNP) level
- Chest x-ray
- Echocardiogram
- Pulmonary artery pressure catheterization

Management

- Primary goal in managing heart failure is to maintain cardiac output.
- Secondary goal is to decrease venous (capillary) pressure to limit edema.
- Diuretics (furosemide): Aimed at controlling fluid retention.
- Beta blockers (metoprolol): Aimed at reducing cardiac workload.
- Nitrates (NTG, nitroprusside): Aimed at enhancing myocardial contractility.
- Inotropes (dobutamine): Aimed at enhancing myocardial contractility.

Abdominal Aortic Aneurysm (AAA)

AAA is a localized, chronic abnormal dilation of an artery located between the renal and iliac arteries, having a diameter at least 1.5 times that of the expected diameter with a natural history toward enlargement and rupture.

Pathophysiology

There are just theories about the pathology of AAA because the etiology is not completely understood. Theories suggest that atherosclerosis and destruction of elastin and collagen fibers in the vessel walls contribute to the development.

Pathophysiology for Atherosclerosis

Fatty streaks deposited in arterial intima → stimulates inflammatory response that causes proliferation → proliferation causes blood vessel to form fibrous capillaries → deposits build up as atheromas or plaques → plaques pile up, obstructing the blood flow → outpouching of abdominal aneurysm.

Pathophysiology Involvement with Elastin and Collagen

Media thins → decrease in elastin fibers in vessel walls → collagen weakens → leads to aneurysm growth → outpouching of abdominal aorta

Clinical Presentation

AAA may present as asymptomatic or symptomatic. When asymptomatic, look for a pulsatile, periumbilical mass with or without a bruit. When symptomatic, symptoms include:

- Early satiety
- Nausea
- Vomiting
- Gastrointestinal bleeding
- Back pain
- Lower extremity ischemia
- Venous thrombosis
- Flank/groin pain

AAA can also mimic:

- UTI infection
- Renal obstruction
- Ruptured disc
- Diverticulitis
- Pancreatitis
- Upper gastrointestinal hemorrhage
- Abdominal neoplasm
- Peptic ulcer perforation

Diagnostic Tests

- Abdominal ultrasound (first line of diagnostic testing)
- CT scan of the abdomen
- Abdominal x-ray
- Aortogram

Management

- Administer beta blocker to lower arterial pressure to the lowest SBP (120 mm Hg or less).
- May use newer alpha-beta-blocker labetalol (Trandate) in place of nitroprusside and a beta blocker; do not give direct vasodilators such as hydralazine.

Postoperative Management

- Goal of postoperative care is to reduce afterload and pressure at the repair site.
- Administer IV nitroprusside with esmolol (Brevibloc) or labetalol (Trandate) and titrate the dosage to keep systolic BP below 120 mm Hg as ordered.
- Starting immediately after surgery, continuously monitor the patient's neurological status, cardiac rhythm, RR, hemodynamics, urine output, core body temperature, fluid and electrolyte imbalance.
- Provide analgesia.
- Monitor for acute renal failure, ischemic colitis, spinal cord ischemia, and aorto-enteric fistula.
- Assess patient's gastrointestinal function.
- Report urine output less than 0.5 mL/kg/hr, which indicates dehydration, volume deficit, or decreased renal function.

Aortic Dissection

Aortic dissection is a tear (without hematoma or an intramural hematoma) in the aortic wall, causing a longitudinal separation between the intima and adventitia layers resulting in a diversion of blood flow from its normal arterial pathway. Aortic dissection requires emergent surgery.

Pathophysiology

Tear in aorta intima → blood flows into subintimal region → pulsatile pressure creates a false channel between intimal and medial layers of aorta → intimal and medial layer is separated → circulatory volume decreases → channel expands and creates either an expanding mass or a hematoma (from blood coagulating) → lumen narrows and obstructs blood flow, cardiac output decreases → results in end-organ failure, also diverted blood can pool around heart, resulting in cardiac tamponade.

Clinical Presentation

Consider acute phase if diagnosed within first 2 weeks of onset of pain.

Presenting Symptoms
- Mimics inferior wall MI
- CHF
- CVAP
- Standard type A aortic dissection: Severe chest pain, sometimes sharp
- Standard type B dissection: Severe chest pain radiating to the back; described as "ripping or tearing" pain
- Pain can shift to the abdomen
- Increasing restlessness (sign of extending dissection)
- Decrease in urine output

Diagnostic Tests

- Chest x-ray: Shows widening mediastinum
- ECG
- Transthoracic echocardiogram
- Transesophageal echocardiogram
- CT scan
- Aortography
- MRI

Management

- Measure BP in both arms. Monitor HR, RR, and pain level.
- Perform frequent peripheral pulse checks, ankle brachial index measurements, and neurological assessments.
- Administer beta blockers as first line of treatment; if hypertensive → give nitroprusside IV.
- Plan for emergency surgery.

Pericardial Effusion

Pericardial effusion is the abnormal accumulation of more than 50 mL of fluid (normal: 15–50 mL to serve as lubricant for the visceral and parietal layers of pericardium) in the pericardial sac, which may lead to noncompression of the heart, which interferes with heart function.

Pathophysiology

Causes: chest trauma, accidents, stab wounds, gun shot wounds, rupture of tumors, obstruction of lymphatic or venous flow → accumulate blood in the pericardial sac → ↑ pressure → compresses or does not compress the heart.

Clinical Manifestations

Pericardial effusion can be asymptomatic with up to 2 L accumulated fluid in the pericardial sac.

- Complaints of dull, constant ache in the left side of the chest with symptoms of cardiac compression.
- Muffled heart sounds.
- May or may not present with pericardial friction.
- Dullness of percussion of the left lung over the angle of scapula (Ewart's sign).
- ECG shows ↓ voltage of complexes.

Diagnostic Tests

- Echocardiogram

Management

- Pain management.
- Pericardiocentesis performed by a physician.
- Position changes decrease SOB.

- Wound care after pericardiocentesis, care of pericardial catheters.
- Frequent assessments of VS, pulses, LOC, respiratory status, skin and temperature changes, intake and output.
- Prevent cardiac tamponade.

Cardiac Surgeries

Coronary Artery Bypass Graft (CABG)

CABG is an open-heart surgical procedure in which a blood vessel from another part of the body, usually the saphenous vein from the leg, is grafted below the occluded coronary artery so that blood can bypass the blockage.

Pathophysiology

Surgery is performed on those patients with coronary artery disease, causing blockage to the coronary arteries. Fatty streaks deposited in arterial intima stimulates an inflammatory response that causes proliferation. Proliferation causes blood vessels to form fibrous caps, and deposits build up as atheromas or plaques. Plaques pile up obstructing the blood flow.

Clinical Manifestations

Ischemia: if ischemic episode lasts long enough can cause death to myocardial cells → MI, angina, chest pain, somatic and visceral pain and discomfort. Atrial fibrillation common complication of cardiac surgery.

Diagnostic Tests

- Health history
- Exercise treadmill testing
- Gated SPECT imaging
- Echocardiography
- Electron Beam Computed Tomography (EBCT)
- Lab work: lipid profile

Postoperative Care

- Common postop care includes maintaining airway patency and monitoring the patient's pulmonary status, vital signs, intake and output.
- Perform peripheral and neurovascular assessments hourly for first 8 hours.

- Monitor neurological status.
- Titrate drugs: vasopressor and inotropes to optimize cardiac function and BP.
- Monitor chest tube drainage and record amount.
- Watch for signs of bleeding and monitor hemoglobin and hematocrit every 4 hours.
- Monitor patient's pain and medicate as needed.

Coronary Stenting/Percutaneous Coronary Intervention

Percutaneous coronary intervention (PCI) is a common intervention for angina. In a catheterization lab, a catheter equipped with an inflatable balloon tip is inserted into the appropriate coronary artery. When the lesion is located, the catheter is passed through the lesion, the balloon is inflated, and the atherosclerotic plaque is compressed, resulting in vessel dilatation. Intracoronary stents are usually inserted during PCI. Stents are used to treat abrupt or threatened abrupt closure or restenosis following PCI.

Procedure
Stents are expandable meshlike structures designed to maintain vessel patency by compressing the arterial walls and resisting vasoconstriction. Stents are carefully placed over the angioplasty site to hold the vessel open.

Clinical Presentation
- Atypical or typical chest pain
- SOB
- Dyspnea
- Symptoms of angina

Diagnostic Tests
- ECG
- Echocardiogram
- Chest x-ray
- Lab tests: cardiac markers

Management of Clinical Condition
- Administer antiplatelet agents (aspirin, ticlopidine, clopidogrel).
- Administer IV infusion of glycoprotein IIb IIIa inhibitors (eptifibatide).

- Monitor for signs and symptoms of bleeding at catheter site.
- Monitor for chest pain.

Stent Insertion

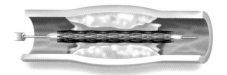

Stent Inflation and Expansion

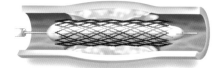

Balloon Removal and Stent Implantation

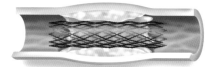

Cardiac Valve Replacement

Clinical conditions that require a surgical procedure to replace the valve with either a mechanical valve or a porcine valve include:

- Acquired valvular dysfunction
- Mitral valve stenosis
- Mitral valve regurgitation
- Mitral valve prolapse
- Aortic stenosis
- Aortic regurgitation

The surgical procedure is the same as open-heart surgery except the heart is not bypassed, only the valve is replaced.

Pathophysiology

Mitral stenosis: Usually results from rheumatic fever (which can cause valve thickening), atrial myxoma (tumor), calcium accumulation, or thrombus formation → valve becomes stiff. The valve opening narrows → prevention of normal blood flow from left atrium to left ventricle → pulmonary congestion → right-sided heart failure.

- Mitral valve regurgitation: Fibrotic and calcific changes prevent mitral valve from closing completely during systole → incomplete closure of the valve → backflow of blood into left atrium when left ventricle contracts → increased volume ejection with next systole → increased pressure → left ventricular hypertrophy.
- Mitral valve prolapse: The valvular leaflets enlarge and prolapse into left atrium during systole → usually benign but may lead to mitral valve regurgitation.
- Aortic stenosis: Aortic valve orifice narrows and obstructs left ventricle outflow during systole → increased resistance to ejection or afterload → ventricular hypertrophy.
- Aortic regurgitation: Aortic valve leaflets do not close properly → regurgitation of aortic blood back into ventricle during diastole → left ventricular hypertrophy.

Clinical Presentation

- **Mitral stenosis:** Fatigue, dyspnea on exertion, orthopnea, paroxysmal nocturnal dyspnea, hemoptysis, hepatomegaly, JVD, pitting edema, atrial fibrillation, apical diastolic murmur.
- **Mitral valve regurgitation:** Fatigue, dyspnea on exertion, orthopnea, palpitations, atrial fibrillation, JVD, pitting edema, high-pitched holosystolic murmur.
- **Mitral valve prolapse:** Atypical chest pain, dizziness, syncope, palpitations, atrial tachycardia, ventricular tachycardia, systolic click.
- **Aortic stenosis:** Dyspnea on exertion, angina, syncope on exertion, fatigue, orthopnea, paroxysmal nocturnal dyspnea, harsh systolic crescendo-decrescendo murmur.
- **Aortic insufficiency:** Palpitations, dyspnea, orthopnea, paroxysmal nocturnal dyspnea, fatigue, angina, sinus tachycardia, blowing decrescendo diastolic murmur.

Diagnostic Tests

- Echocardiogram
- ECG
- Cardiac angiogram
- Exercise tolerance test

Management

- Routine postoperative care: maintain airway patency, monitor pulmonary status.
- Monitor vital signs and intake and output.
- Perform peripheral and neurovascular assessments hourly for first 8 hours after surgery.
- Monitor neurological status for first 8 hours postoperatively.
- Titrate medications, pressors and inotropes to optimize cardiac function and BP.
- Monitor chest tube drainage.
- Watch for signs of bleeding by monitoring hgb and hct every 4 hours.
- Monitor for pain.
- Start on anticoagulation therapy when approved by cardiac surgeon.

Cardiac Transplant

Cardiac transplant is a surgical procedure to remove a diseased heart and replace it with a healthy donor heart.

Causes That Lead to Cardiac Transplant

End-stage heart disease includes congenital heart disease (single ventricle physiology, coronary sinusoids), cardiomyopathy (primary: idiopathic, familial, secondary pregnancy, drug-induced), and acquired heart disease (valvular disease).

Criteria for Heart Transplant
- CHF
- CAD with intractable angina symptoms,
- Ventricular dysrhythmias unresponsive to medical/surgery therapy
- Primary cardiac tumors with no evidence of spread to other body systems

Diagnostic Tests Prior to Transplantation
- Echocardiogram
- Right heart catheterization
- Pulmonary function tests
- Exercise treadmill test
- Abdominal ultrasound
- Chest x-rays
- Coronary angiogram
- Cardiac biopsy
- Chromosome testing
- Lab tests: chemistries, CBC, human leukocyte antigens (HLA) antibody screening, viral antibody screening (HIV, cytomegalovirus, herpes virus, varicella, Epstein- Barr)

Postoperative Care
- Admit to Cardio Thoracic ICU, 24–48 hours on ventilator until anesthesia cleared from system.
- Foley catheter to gravity, monitor output closely.
- Daily chest x-ray.
- Monitor chest tube sites and drainage (generally will have 2–3 chest tubes in place).

- Pulmonary toilet measures hourly, once extubated.
- Perform and document complete nursing assessments frequently during first 12–24 hours after surgery.
- Watch for signs and symptoms of bleeding.
- Treat dysrhythmias.
- Prevention of right-sided heart failure.
- Watch for early signs of rejection, infection, immunosuppressive issues.
- Monitor for signs of drug toxicity.
- ICU care for about 3–5 days post-op.
- Treatment of rejection: treated with increased doses of cyclosporine, azathioprine, high-dose corticosteroids, prednisone, monoclonal antibodies or polyclonal antibodies.
- Highest risk for infection: 1 week post-op.

Signs and Symptoms of Rejection

- Low-grade fever
- Fatigue
- SOB
- Peripheral edema
- Pulmonary crackles
- Pericardial friction rub
- Arrhythmias
- Decreased ECG voltage
- Increased JVD
- Hypotension
- Cardiac enlargement on x-ray
- Vascular degeneration
- Tachycardia
- Fatigue
- Palpitations
- Nausea and vomiting

Other Complications

- Infection
- CAD

Carotid Endarterectomy (CE)

CE is a surgical procedure to remove plaque material from inside the carotid artery, improving the carotid luminal diameter, allowing adequate blood flow, therefore preventing stroke. The procedure is indicated in symptomatic patients with carotid-territory TIA or minor strokes who have carotid artery stenosis of 70%–99%.

Pathophysiology of the Disease Process Leading to CE
Surgery is performed on patients with symptomatic carotid artery stenosis. Fatty streaks are deposited in arterial intima → stimulates inflammatory response that causes proliferation → blood vessels forming fibrous caps → deposit buildup as atheromas or plaques → plaques build up causing blood flow obstruction.

Clinical Presentation
- Signs and symptoms of TIA or stroke
- Dizziness
- Lightheadedness

Diagnostic Tests
- Ultrasound of carotid artery
- Magnetic resonance angiography (MRA)
- Contrast enhanced MRA (CEMRA)
- Intra-arterial angiography (IAA)

Management of Clinical Condition
- Assess surgical site for bleeding.
- Perform frequent neurological checks.
- Administer antihypertensive medications.
- Administer statins.
- Administer antiplatelet agents.
- Administer aspirin (81–325 mg) before and after surgery.

Infections of the Heart

Endocarditis

Endocarditis is the inflammation of the inner most layer of the heart. It can include the heart valves, chordae tendinea, cardiac septum or the lining of the chambers. It is caused typically by bacterial infections (*Streptococcus viridans* or *Staphylococcus aureus*).

Pathophysiology

Microbe invades the valve leaflets → infection occurs causing valve leaflets to be deformed

Clinical Presentation

Endocarditis presents as:

- Acute onset of fever
- Chills
- Night sweats
- Anorexia
- Myalgia
- Arthralgia
- Extreme fatigue and malaise
- Nausea and vomiting
- Headache
- Weight loss
- SOB
- Chest pain
- Abdominal pain
- Confusion
- Pain in the muscles, joints, and back

Be suspicious if petechiae appears on the conjunctiva, neck, anterior chest, abdomen, or oral mucosa. Look for Janeway lesions (nontender macule) on patient's palms and soles, Osler's nodes (tender, erythematous, raised nodules) on fingers and toe pads, and splinter hemorrhages under fingernails.

Diagnostic Tests

- Transthoracic echocardiogram
- Abdominal computed tomography (CT) or MRI
- Positive blood cultures

Management

- Antibiotic prophylaxis before certain invasive procedures.
- Priorities include supporting cardiac function, eradicating the infection, and preventing complications, such as systemic embolization and heart failure.
- Do not give anticoagulants because of risk of intracerebral hemorrhage.

Pericarditis

Pericarditis is inflammation of pericardium that can cause fluid to accumulate in the pericardial space due to idiopathic causes, infection, cardiac complications, autoimmune reactions, certain drugs, or trauma.

Pathophysiology

Primary illness of medical or surgical disorder can be the etiology → pericardium becomes inflamed → can lead to excess fluid accumulation or increased pressure on the heart leading to tamponade.

Clinical Presentation

Sharp, constant chest pain that is located in the midchest (retrosternal) is the most common symptom. A hallmark sign of pericarditis is if the patient leans forward while sitting to relieve chest pain. Pain may radiate to the neck, shoulders, and back; radiation to the ridge of the left trapezius muscle is specific for pericarditis.

Depending on the cause, patient may also have fever, malaise, tachypnea, and tachycardia. Pericardial friction rub, heard in the lower sternal border, is the most important physical sign.

Diagnostic Tests

- ECG
- Echocardiogram
- Chest x-ray

- Lab work: cardiac markers
- Complete blood count
- Urinalysis
- Transesophageal echocardiogram (TEE)

Management
- NSAIDs may be used for up to 2 weeks.
- Monitor for cardiac tamponade.
- More severe pain can be controlled with morphine.
- If cause is infectious, antibiotics or antifungal drugs may be administered.
- Treatment: Antibiotics specific to the pathogen for at least 6 weeks.
- If a pericardiectomy is performed, continue assessments of VS, lab work, and the appearance of wounds and insertion sites of invasive lines.
- Monitor temperature and cardiac rhythm, assess for heart murmurs.
- Perform neurological assessments, inspect skin surfaces, and monitor drug peaks and troughs, and urine output.

Pacemakers/AICD

There are three types of pacemakers:

- Transcutaneous (external)
- Percutaneous
- Permanent

Transcutaneous Pacemakers

Transcutaneous pacemakers are used for noninvasive temporary pacing, accomplished through the application of two large external electrodes. The electrodes are attached to an external pulse generator, which can operate on alternating current or battery. The generator emits electrical pulses, which are transmitted through the electrodes and then transcutaneously to stimulate ventricular depolarization when the patient's heart rate is slower than the rate set on the pacemaker. Used as an emergency measure, a transcutaneous pacemaker should be used for 48–72 hours only. Electrodes should be changed every 24 hours minimally.

Percutaneous Pacemakers

Percutaneous pacemakers are for invasive temporary pacing. An invasive temporary pacemaker system consists of an external battery pulse generator and pacing electrodes, or lead wires. These wires attach to the generator on one end and are in contact with the heart on the other end. Electrical pulses, or stimuli, are emitted from the negative terminal or the generator, flow through a lead wire and stimulate the cardiac cells to depolarize.

Permanent Pacemakers

Permanent pacing is performed for the resolution of nontemporary conduction disorders, including complete heart block and sick sinus syndrome. Permanent pacemakers are usually powered by a lithium battery and have an average life span of 10 years.

Automatic Implantable Cardioverter Device (AICD)

AICD is indicated for the patient who has experienced one or more episodes of spontaneous sustained ventricular tachycardia (VT) or ventricular fibrillation (VF) unrelated to MI or other causes amendable to correction.

Cardiac Tamponade

Cardiac tamponade is excessive fluid or blood from the heart in the pericardial space that accumulates pressure in the pericardial sac and affects the heart's function.

Pathophysiology

Causes: accidents, stab wounds, gun shot wounds, rupture of tumors, obstruction of lymphatic or venous flow → accumulate blood in the pericardial sac → ↑ venous pressure → compress all four chambers of the heart → RA and RV are compressed → ↓ RA filling during diastole → ↓ venous blood returns to RA

$\rightarrow$ ↑ venous pressure $\rightarrow$ JVD, edema, hepatomegaly, ↑ DBP $\rightarrow$ continued compression of the heart $\rightarrow$ ↓ diastolic filling of ventricles $\rightarrow$ ↓ SV, ↓ CO, ↓ tissue perfusion $\rightarrow$ body attempts to increase blood volume, increase SV $\rightarrow$ ↑ workload of the heart $\rightarrow$ body compensation $\rightarrow$ tachycardia $\rightarrow$ all of these complications last for a limited amount of time $\rightarrow$ shock, cardiac arrest, or death if not immediately corrected.

Clinical Manifestations

First Signs
- Anxiety and restlessness
- Cool, diaphoretic skin

Classic Signs
- Beck's triad: muffled heart sounds, increased JVD, and hypotension
- Narrow pulse pressure (SBP and DBP)
- Tachycardia
- Weak, thready pulse

Late Signs
- Pulsus paradoxus (↓ SBP of more than 10 mm Hg on inspiration)
- Electrical alternans (alternating levels of voltage in the P waves and QRS complexes in all leads and may occur in T waves)

Diagnostic Tests

- Chest x-ray
- Echocardiogram

Management

- Call MD stat.
- Obtain Stat 2-D echocardiogram.
- Obtain Stat chest x-ray.
- Obtain Stat lab work.
- MD to place PA catheter.
- Place patient in supine position, HOB elevated 30°–60°.
- Administer O_2.
- Give sedatives, morphine for chest pain.

- Obtain ECG.
- If on mechanical ventilation: No positive pressure used.
- Inotropic drugs on standby.
- Blood, plasma, volume expander on hand.

ACLS Algorithms: Cardiac/Respiratory Arrest

Ventricular Fibrillation (VF) or Pulseless Ventricular Tachycardia (VT)

- **Shock:** Biphasic: 200 J; monophasic: 360 J. Reassess rhythm.
- **CPR:** Immediately perform 5 cycles of CPR (should last about 2 min).
- **Epinephrine:** 1 mg IV or IO (2 to 2.5 mg, endotracheal tube) every 3–5 min or **Vasopressin:** 40 units IV or IO, one time only. May use to replace 1st or 2nd dose of epinephrine (given without interrupting CPR).
- **Shock:** Biphasic: 200 J; monophasic: 360 J. Reassess rhythm.
- **Consider antiarrhythmics** (given without interrupting CPR):
  - **Amiodarone:** 300 mg IV or IO, may repeat 150 mg in 3–5 min.
  - **Lidocaine:** 1.0–1.5 mg/kg IV or IO, may repeat 0.5 to 0.75 mg/kg q5–10 min, max 3 mg/kg.
  - **Magnesium:** 1–2 g IV or IO for Torsade de Pointes.

Asystole or PEA (Pulseless Electrical Activity)

- Resume CPR for 5 cycles (should last about 2 minutes).
- **Epinephrine:** 1 mg IV or IO (2 to 2.5 mg ET) every 3–5 min or **Vasopressin:** 40 units IV or IO, one time only. May use to replace 1st or 2nd dose of epinephrine (given without interrupting CPR).
- **Atropine:** 1 mg IV (2 to 3 mg endotracheal tube every 3–5 min) (maximum 3 mg) for asystole or bradycardic PEA.

Intra-Aortic Balloon Pump (IABP)

An IABP consists of a 30-cm polyurethane balloon attached to one end of a large bore catheter. The device is inserted into the femoral artery at the groin, either percutaneously or via arteriotomy, with the balloon wrapped tightly around the catheter. Once inserted, the catheter is advanced up the aorta until the tip lies just beyond the origin of the L subclavian artery. When in place, the balloon wrapping is released to allow periodic balloon inflations.

Effects

The intra-aortic balloon is inflated with helium at the onset of each diastolic period, when the aortic valve closes. The balloon is deflated at the onset of ventricular systole, just before aortic valve opens. Inflation of the balloon increases the peak diastolic pressure and displaces blood toward the periphery. Deflation of the balloon decreases the end-diastolic pressure, which reduces impedance to flow when aortic valve opens at onset of systole. This decreases ventricular afterload and promotes stroke volume.

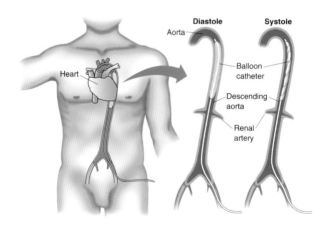

IABP waveforms

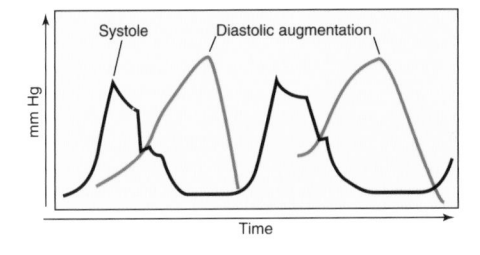

Indications

- Cardiopulmonary bypass
- Cardiac transplant
- AMI with cardiogenic shock
- Acute mitral valve insufficiency
- Unstable angina

Contraindications

- Aortic regurgitation
- Aortic dissection
- Recently placed (within 12 months) prosthetic graft in thoracic aorta

ECGs

12-Lead ECG

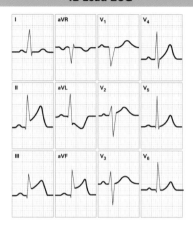

Lead Placement

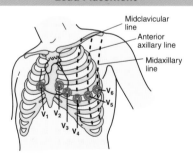

Hemodynamics of Dysrhythmias

Atrial Dysrhythmias

Atrial dysrhythmias are caused by increased automaticity in the atria. The patient may complain of palpitations or "heart racing." Loss of atrial contraction → shortens diastole → loss of atrial kick (25%–30% of C.O.) → ↓ C.O. → ↓ coronary perfusion → ischemic myocardial changes.

Causes
- Amphetamines
- Cocaine
- Decongestants
- Hypokalemia
- Hyperthyroidism
- COPD
- Pericarditis
- Digoxin toxicity
- Hypothermia
- Alcohol intoxication
- Pulmonary edema

Ventricular Dysrhythmias

Ventricular dysrhythmias are caused by increased automaticity in the ventricles. PVCs—patient complains of "heart skipping a beat." This dysrhythmia can lead to bradycardia → ↓ C.O. → ↓ BP and eventually VT, VF, and death.

Bradycardia
Bradycardia is defined as a heart rate less than 60 bpm. ↓HR → ↓ C.O. → ↓ BP → ↓ perfusion to brain, heart, kidneys, lung & skin.

Causes
- Vomiting
- Gagging
- Valsalva maneuver
- ETT suctioning

Symptoms
- Chest pain
- SOB
- Altered mental status

Treatment Considerations
- Atropine
- Epinephrine
- Isoproterenol (Isuprel)
- Pacemaker
- Dopamine if hypotensive

Tachycardia

Tachycardia is defined as a heart rate greater than 100 bpm. $\uparrow\uparrow$ HR can compromise C.O. by $\downarrow$ ventricular filling $\rightarrow$ $\downarrow$ SV $\rightarrow$ $\downarrow$ C.O. $\rightarrow$ $\uparrow$ workload of the heart $\rightarrow$ $\uparrow$ O_2 consumption.

Causes
- Caffeine
- Nicotine
- Pain
- Fever
- Stress
- Anxiety

Symptoms
- Altered LOC
- Chest pain or discomfort
- Palpitations
- SOB
- Diaphoresis
- Hypotension
- Jugular venous distention

Treatment Considerations
- Carotid massage
- Valsalva maneuver
- Cardiovert at 100 J–360 J
- Radiofrequency ablation
- Pacemaker

- If arrhythmia converts to pulseless VT or VF → defibrillate
- Implantable cardioverter defibrillator (ICD), if indicated

Determining Rate and Measurement

To figure out rate (regular rhythms only), you can do one of the following:

Count the number of QRS complexes (regular rhythms only) in a 6-sec strip and multiply by 10.

Irregular rhythms should be counted for an entire minute.

Divide the number of large boxes between two R waves into 300.

Remember the number sequence below and find an R wave that falls on a heavy line. Starting from the next heavy line, count 300, 150, 100, and so forth, and whatever line the next R wave falls on is the heart rate (see below for example).

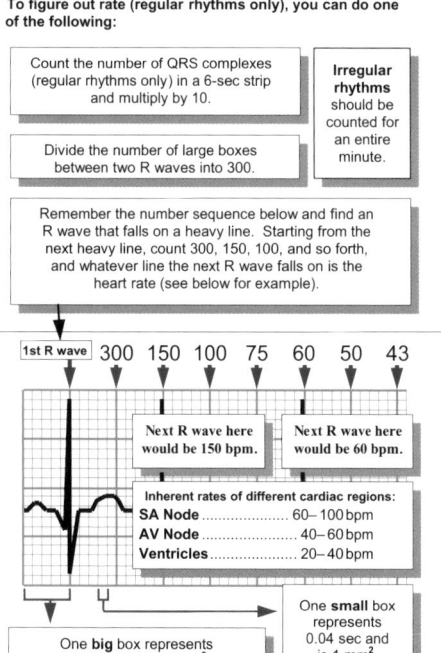

1st R wave   300   150   100   75   60   50   43

Next R wave here would be 150 bpm.

Next R wave here would be 60 bpm.

Inherent rates of different cardiac regions:
SA Node .... 60–100 bpm
AV Node .... 40–60 bpm
Ventricles .... 20–40 bpm

One **big** box represents 0.20 sec and is 5 mm².

One **small** box represents 0.04 sec and is 1 mm².

Normal Cardiac Cycle and Measurements

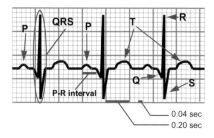

Normal Rate → 60 to 100 bpm
Normal P-R → 0.12 to 0.20 sec
Normal QRS → 0.08 to 0.12 sec
  P wave → atrial depolarization; **QRS** → ventricular **de**polarization;
T wave → ventricular **re**polarization

Quick Guide to Analyzing the ECG

■ Determine the overall rate: <60 bpm → bradycardia, >100 bpm
  → tachycardia.
■ Determine the regularity: Regular or irregular.
  ■ If irregular, is there any pattern?
■ Examine the P waves.
  ■ Is there a P wave before each QRS? Is there more than 1 P wave?
  ■ Are P waves absent?
  ■ What is the configuration of the P wave? Round? Saw toothed?
  ■ Do they look the same?
  ■ Do any occur earlier or later than expected?
  ■ Are any P waves located within the QRS or T wave?
■ Determine the PR interval.
  ■ Is it normal, prolonged, or shortened?
  ■ Can it be measured?
  ■ Is it the same for each beat? Any pattern?

■ Examine the QRS complex.
   ■ Is there a QRS after each P wave?
   ■ Do they look the same?
   ■ Do any occur earlier than expected?
   ■ Is there a pattern to QRS complexes occurring early?

Normal Cardiac Rhythm Parameters	
NSR	• 60 bpm–100 bpm
Bradycardia	• <60 bpm; consider sinus bradycardia, AV block
Tachycardia	• >100 bpm; consider atrial fibrillation, atrial flutter, supraventricular tachycardia, ventricular tachycardia
PR interval	• 0.12–0.20 sec
	• >0.20 sec; consider AV block
	• <0.12 sec; consider junctional rhythm
	• Unable to determine; consider atrial arrhythmia, junctional arrhythmia; examine QRS to determine if ventricular arrhythmia
P wave	• Generally round
	• Saw toothed → Consider atrial flutter
	• Spiked, nonrounded; consider atrial fibrillation or PACs
QRS	• 0.06–0.10 sec
	• Wide, bizarre; consider PVC, VT

Baseline is grossly irregular with no discernible P waves; consider VT
Flat baseline, asystole; begin CPR for either dysrhythmia.

Supraventricular Tachycardia (SVT)

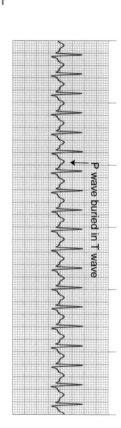

P wave buried in T wave

Rate: 150–250 bpm

Rhythm: Usually regular

PR interval: Unable to determine

P waves: Usually hidden in preceding T wave

QRS: 0.06–0.10 sec, >0.10 sec if conducted through the ventricles

Causes: Nicotine, stress, anxiety, caffeine

Management: Vagal maneuver, adenosine (Adenocard, Adenoscan), amiodarone (Cordarone, Pacerone), diltiazem (Cardizem), cardioversion, propafenone (Rythmol), flecainide (Tambocor)

Atrial Flutter

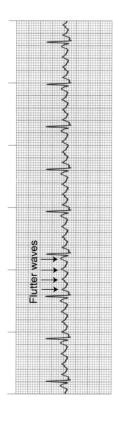

Flutter waves

AV node conducts impulses to the ventricle with varying degrees of block (2:1 → 2 flutter waves:1 QRS; 4:1 → 4 flutter waves: 1 QRS). Seen in coronary artery disease and valvular disease.

- **Atrial rate:** 250–400 bpm
- **PR interval:** Unable to determine
- **Rhythm:** Regular or irregular depending if combination of degrees of block (e.g., 2:1 + 4:1)
- **P waves:** Saw-toothed flutter waves
- **Ventricular rate:** Slow or fast depending on degree of block
- **QRS:** Normal or narrow
- **Management:** Diltiazem; sotalol, propranolol or other beta blockers, digoxin, amiodarone, propafenone, flecainide, magnesium, electrical cardioversion, radiofrequency ablation; anticoagulate

Atrial Fibrillation

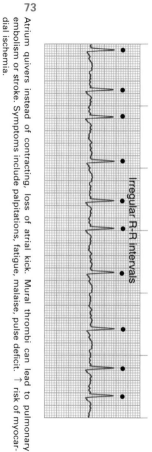

Irregular R-R intervals

Atrium quivers instead of contracting, loss of atrial kick. Mural thrombi can lead to pulmonary embolism or stroke. Symptoms include palpitations, fatigue, malaise, pulse deficit. → risk of myocardial ischemia.

- **Atrial rate:** 400–600 bpm
- **PR interval:** Unable to determine
- **Rhythm:** Irregularly irregular
- **P waves:** None; fibrillatory waves
- **Ventricular rate:** Normal or fast
- **QRS:** Usually narrow
- **Management:** Same as atrial flutter; ibutilide (Corvert) after cardioversion; anticoagulate

Premature Ventricular Contractions (PVC)

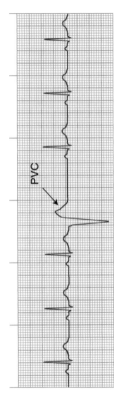

PVC

May be uniform (one ectopic focus or unifocal) or different foci (multifocal).
Patient may complain of lightheadedness, palpitations, heart skipping a beat.

- **P wave:** Absent before PVC
- **Rhythm:** Irregular where PVC occurs
- **QRS:** Wide, bizarre, >0.10 sec; may be followed by compensatory pause
- **Causes:** Healthy persons, caffeine, nicotine, stress, cardiac ischemia or infarction, digoxin toxicity, electrolyte imbalances, hypovolemia, fever, hypokalemia, hypoxia, hypermagnesemia, acid-base imbalance
- **Management:** Correct the cause, amiodarone, lidocaine

Ventricular Tachycardia (VT)

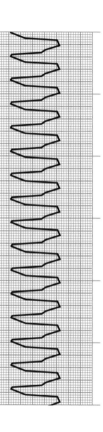

Three or more PVCs together with the same shape and amplitude.
Unstable rhythm. Easily progresses to VF if VT sustained & untreated.
Patient may or may not have a pulse, no BP.

■ **Atrial rate:** Unable to determine; no P waves; no PR interval
■ **Ventricular rate:** 100–250 bpm
■ **Rhythm:** Usually regular
■ **QRS:** Wide & bizarre, >0.10 sec
■ **Management:** Amiodarone, procainamide, lidocaine, sotalol, immediate synchronized cardioversion; pulseless VT is treated the same as VF

Ventricular Fibrillation (VF)

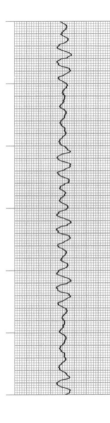

Chaotic pattern. No effective ventricular contraction. No C.O., no pulse, no BP. Brain death occurs within 4–6 min, if untreated.

- **Atrial rate:** Unable to determine; no P waves; no PR interval
- **Ventricular rate:** Fibrillatory waves with no pattern
- **Rhythm:** Irregular
- **Management:** Amiodarone, procainamide, lidocaine, magnesium sulfate, immediate defibrillation at 200 J–360 J; CPR with epinephrine, vasopressin & sodium bicarbonate; intubate, IV access if none present, induce mild hypothermia 32°C–34°C (89.6°F–93.2°F)

First-Degree AV Block

Problem in the conduction system. May progress to more severe block. Patient usually has no symptoms & no hemodynamic changes.

- ■ **P wave:** Present, before each QRS
- ■ **Rhythm:** Regular
- ■ **PR interval:** >0.12 sec
- ■ **QRS:** Normal
- ■ **Management:** Correct the cause, close monitoring, usually benign

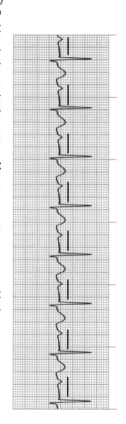

Second-Degree AV Block—Mobitz I or Wenckebach Phenomenon

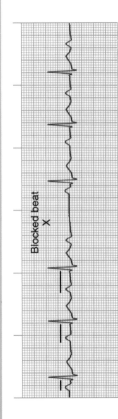

Blocked beat
X

Almost always temporary. If bradycardia → ↓ C.O. Resolves when underlying condition corrected (MI, CAD, drug induced: beta blockers, calcium channel blockers).

- **P wave:** Present until one P wave is blocked with no resultant QRS
- **Rhythm:** Irregular
- **PR interval:** Gets progressively longer until a QRS is dropped
- **QRS:** Normal
- **Management:** Correct the underlying cause, atropine, temporary pacemaker

Second-Degree AV Block—Mobitz II

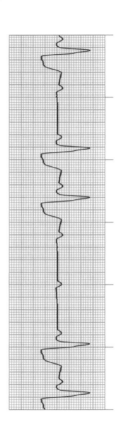

Problem with bundle of His or bundle branches.

Bradycardia → ↓ C.O. → ↓ BP. Patient symptomatic.

May progress to more serious block.

- **P wave:** Present but atrial rate > ventricular rate
  - Conduction of P waves:QRS complexes in 2:1, 3:1 or 4:1 manner
- **Rhythm:** Regular
- **PR interval:** Normal if P wave followed by QRS
- **QRS:** Normal but QRS periodically missing, sometimes wide
- **Management:** Atropine for bradycardia, isoproterenol if very slow rate, pacemaker

Third-Degree AV Block—Complete Heart Block

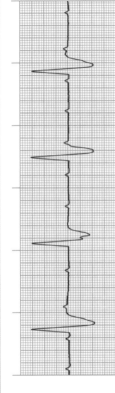

Loss of synchrony between atrial and ventricular contractions.

Potentially life-threatening.

Bradycardia → ↓↓ C.O. → ↓ BP. Patient symptomatic.

Digoxin toxicity a frequent cause.

- **P wave:** Present but atrial rate > ventricular rate
  - Conduction of P waves in no relation to QRS complexes
- **Rhythm:** Regular atrial rate and ventricular rate
- **PR interval:** No relation of P waves to QRS complexes
- **QRS:** Usually wide
- **Management:** Atropine for bradycardia, isoproterenol, pacemaker

Respiratory Disorders

Adult Respiratory Distress Syndrome (ARDS)

ARDS is defined as noncardiogenic pulmonary edema characterized by severe refractory hypoxemic respiratory failure and decreased pulmonary compliance.

Pathophysiology

↑ capillary/alveolar membrane permeability → interstitial & alveolar leak → right-to-left intrapulmonary shunting → severe and refractory hypoxemia, metabolic acidosis. Inactivation of surfactant → alveolar atelectasis, ↓ lung compliance → hypoventilation and hypercapnia.

Clinical Presentation

Symptoms of ARDS occur within 24 to 48 hours of cause and include:

- Increased respiratory rate, increased work of breathing, dyspnea, cyanosis
- Crackles, rhonchi or wheezes, dry cough
- Intercostal and suprasternal retraction, retrosternal discomfort
- Agitation, restlessness, anxiety, confusion
- Diaphoresis
- Abdominal paradox
- Increased pressure to ventilate
    - Hypoxemia refractory to increased fractional concentration of oxygen in inspired gas (FIO_2)
- Increased peak inspiratory pressure
- Decreased lung volume, decreased functional residual capacity, low ventilation/perfusion (V/Q) ratio
- Pulmonary capillary wedge pressure (PCWP) <18 mm Hg and/or no evidence of CHF or left atrial hypertension
- Acute respiratory alkalosis initially, which may progress to respiratory acidosis
- Worsening arterial blood gases (ABGs) with increased FIO_2, increased crackles
    - Worsening partial pressure of arterial oxygen (PaO_2)/FIO_2 (P/F) ratio
- Diffuse bilateral pulmonary infiltrates on chest x-ray (CXR) indicates "whiteout"
- Fluid and electrolyte problems

Diagnostic Tests

- Arterial and venous blood gases
- Mixed venous oxygen saturation
- Continuous oxygenation monitoring via pulse oximetry
- Pulmonary function tests
- Pulmonary artery catheter
- Serial CXRs
- Chest computed tomography (CT)
- CBC, metabolic panel, serum lactate (lactic acid)

Management

- Treat underlying cause.
- Administer O_2 mask or mechanical ventilation with positive end-expiratory pressure (PEEP) and high FIO_2. Consider oscillator ventilator—used when difficulty oxygenating a patient on conventional setting because of poor lung compliance (required neuromuscular blockade).
- Refer to basics: mechanical ventilation, blood gases p. 6 and p. 2.
- Provide continuous arteriovenous hemofiltration (CAVH).
- Maintain hemodynamic stability.
- Administer glucocorticosteroids.
- Administer surfactant therapy.
- Place patient in prone position.
- Administer diuretic; fluid management.
- Provide sedation or therapeutic paralysis if necessary.
- Provide pain control.
- Provide nutritional support.
- Cluster activities to decrease fatigue.
- Investigational management of ARDS includes inhaled nitrous oxide, liquid ventilation, ECMO, alveolar surfactant, and vasodilators.

Extracorporeal Membrane Oxygenation (ECMO)

ECMO is a modified form of cardiorespiratory bypass. It provides oxygenation and pulmonary support for patients in severe respiratory failure, particularly ARDS. Its purpose is to avoid high oxygen concentrations and high peak inspiratory pressures, PEEP, and tidal volume, while allowing the lung to rest and heal.

Venovenous (VV) ECMO

The right internal jugular, saphenous, common iliac, or femoral veins are cannulated. The patient's blood is circulated through a membrane oxygenator in which O_2 is infused and CO_2 removed. ECMO can compensate for approximately 70% of the patient's gas exchange requirements.

Functional oxygen saturation (SpO_2) and CO_2 are monitored continuously to maintain values of 50%–80% and 35–45 mm Hg, respectively.

Complications include infections and sepsis, bleeding, disseminated intravascular coagulation (DIC) and intracranial bleeding, air emboli, renal failure, decubitus ulcers, and heparin-induced thrombocytopenia. Nursing care is aimed toward preventing complications.

Shunting

Anatomic shunt is defined as the diversion of blood flow from the right side of the heart directly into the left side of the heart without coming into contact with the alveoli.

Physiologic shunt (capillary shunt; or right-to-left shunt) is defined as the flow of blood from the right side of the heart, through the lungs, and into the left side of the heart without taking part in alveolar and capillary diffusion. Pulmonary blood perfuses completely unventilated alveoli.

Absolute shunt (true shunt) is defined as a combination of the anatomic and capillary shunt, and is generally refractory to oxygen therapy. The V/Q ratio expresses the relationship of alveolar ventilation to pulmonary capillary perfusion:

- Decreased ventilation plus increased perfusion represents a low V/Q ratio.
- Increased ventilation plus decreased perfusion represents a high V/Q ratio.

Diagnostic Tests
- Alveolar-arterial (A-a) gradient (PaO_2/PaO_2)
  - PAO_2 represents the partial pressure of alveolar O_2 (mm Hg).
  - PaO_2 represents the partial pressure of arterial O_2 (mm Hg).
  - Value is used to calculate the percentage of the estimated shunt.
  - Value represents the difference between the alveolar and arterial oxygen tension.
  - Normal A-a gradient value <15 mm Hg.
  - Value is increased in atrial or ventricular septal defects, pulmonary edema, ARDS, pneumothorax, and V/Q mismatch.

- a/A ratio (PaO_2/PAO_2).
  - If ratio <0.60, shunt is worsening.
- Estimation of shunt using PaO_2/FIO_2 (P/F) ratio:
  - P/F ratio 500 indicates a 5% shunt.
  - P/F ratio 300 indicates a 15% shunt.
  - P/F ratio 200 indicates a 20% shunt.

Ventilator-Assisted Pneumonia (VAP)

VAP is an airway infection that develops more than 48 hours after the patient is intubated. It is associated with increased mortality, prolonged time spent on a ventilator, and increased length of ICU/hospital stay.

Pathophysiology
VAP is usually caused by gram-negative bacilli or *Staphylococcus aureus* via microaspiration of bacteria that colonize the oropharynx and upper airways or bacteria that form a biofilm on or within an endotracheal tube (ETT). The presence of an ETT also impairs cough and mucociliary clearance. Suctioning also contributes to VAP.

Clinical Presentation
VAP presents with:

- Increased RR, HR, and temperature (>38.3°C or 101°F)
- Increased WBC (>10,000/mm^3)
- Increased purulent tracheal secretions
- Crackles
- Worsening oxygenation, hypoxemia, PaO_2/FIO_2 changes

Diagnostic Tests
- CXR shows new or persistent infiltrate
- Tracheal aspirate and blood cultures
- Clinical Pulmonary Infection Score (CPIS) >6
- Bronchoscopy or bronchoalveolar lavage

Management
- Monitor CXR and amount and color of tracheal secretions.
- Give IV antibacterials to which the known causative bacteria are sensitive. Consider:
  - Piperacillin/tazobactam (Zosyn)
  - Gentamicin (Garamycin)

- Tobramycin (Nebcin)
- Vancomycin (Vancocin)
- Ceftazidime (Fortax, Ceptaz)
- Levofloxacin (Levaquin)
- Imipenem/cilastatin (Primaxin)
- Linezolid (Zyvox)
- Ticarcillin (Ticar)
- Daptomycin (Cubicin)
- Ticarcillin (Ticar)
- Ciprofloxacin (Cipro)
- Amikacin (Amikin)
- Aztreonam (Azactam)

Evidence-Based Practice Guidelines to Prevent VAP (Ventilator Bundle):

- Elevate head of bed 30–45 degrees.
- Provide "sedation vacations": Decrease amount and frequency of sedation.
- Assess readiness to extubate and extubate as soon as possible.
- Provide peptic ulcer disease prophylaxis with H_2-receptor inhibitors.
- Provide deep venous thrombosis prophylaxis.
- Use meticulous hand hygiene, use gloves appropriately.
- Use meticulous sterile technique when appropriate.
- Use a continuous aspiration of subglottic secretion (CASS) ETT.
- Provide meticulous oral care every 12 hours, including brushing the teeth with a soft toothbrush, tap water, and toothpaste for 1–2 minutes; brushing the tongue; and applying lip balm and moisturizing swabs. Follow with 0.5 oz of 0.12% chlorhexidine gluconate rinse to tooth enamel, gums, and posterior oropharynx.
- Eliminate routine saline bronchial lavage during ETT suctioning.
- Use continuous lateral rotation therapy (CLRT).
- Drain condensation in ventilator tubing down and away from patient.
- Suction every 4 hours and prn. Replace all suction equipment every 24 hours.
- Feeding tubes should be placed beyond the pylorus of the stomach.
- Discontinue mechanical ventilation as soon as possible. Consider bilevel positive airway pressure (BiPAP) and continuous positive airway pressure (CPAP).

Hospital-Acquired Pneumonia Risk Index †				
Factor		Points	Patient A	Patient B
Temperature (°C)	$\geq$36.5 and $\leq$38.4	0		
	$\geq$38.5 and $\leq$8.9	1		
	$\geq$9 and $\leq$36	2		
Blood leukocytes, µL	$\geq$4,000 and $\leq$11,000	0		
	<4,000 or >11,000	1		
Band forms	$\geq$50%	1		
Tracheal secretions	None	0		
	Nonpurulent	1		
	Purulent	2		
Oxygenation: PaO_2/FIO_2, mm Hg	>240 or ARDS	0		
	$\leq$240 and no ARDS	2		
Pulmonary radiography:	No infiltrate	0		
	Diffuse (or patchy) infiltrate	1		
	Localized infiltrate	2		
Progression of infiltrate*:	None	0		
Progression (heart failure and ARDS excluded)		2		
Growth of pathogenic bacteria on tracheal aspirate culture*:	No, rare, or light growth	0		
	Moderate or heavy growth	1		
	Same bacteria as on Gram stain	1		
Total				

PaO_2/FIO_2 = ratio of arterial O_2 pressure to fraction of inspired O_2; ARDS = acute respiratory distress syndrome.
*Criteria applicable 72 hours after initial diagnosis.
Score >6 suggests hospital-acquired pneumonia.
Score <6 suggests alternative process.
†Adapted from Singh N, Rogers P, Atwood CW, et al: Short-course empiric antibiotic therapy for patients with pulmonary infiltrates in the intensive care unit. *American Journal of Respiratory and Critical Care Medicine* 162:505–511, 2000 In Beers, MH: The Merck Manual, 18th edition.

Community-Acquired Pneumonia (CAP)

CAP is pneumonia or inflammation of the lung parenchyma that develops in the community setting or within 48 hours of hospitalization. There are two types of CAP:

- **Typical or bacterial:** Infection by bacteria in the alveoli that cause inflammation.
- **Atypical or nonbacterial:** "Patchy" inflammatory change in the alveolar sputum and the interstitium of the lungs with less severe symptoms than typical pneumonia.

Pathophysiology
Bacteria (*Streptococcus pneumoniae, Haemophilus influenzae, Staphylococcus aureus*) → aspirated to lung → trapped by mucus producing cells → alveolar macrophages fail → activation of inflammatory mediators, cellular inflation, immune activation → damage bronchial mucous membrane and alveocapillary membrane → fill acini and terminal bronchioles with infectious debris and exudates → edema.

Clinical Presentation
CAP presents with:

- Rapidly rising temperature (101°F–105°F or 38.5°C–40.5°C)
- Chest tightness or discomfort
- Diaphoresis, chills, general malaise
- Tachycardia
- Tachypnea (25–45 breaths/min), shortness of breath (SOB), dyspnea
- Cough with or without sputum

- Inspiratory and expiratory crackles
- Diminished breath sounds
- Hypoxia

Diagnostic Tests
- CXR
- Sputum and blood cultures
- CBC, erythrocyte sedimentation rate (ESR)
- ABGs or O_2 saturation

Management
- Monitor CXR and amount and color of tracheal secretions.
- Provide oxygenation and ventilation: O_2 by cannula/mask, mechanical ventilation. Assess oxygenation status by ABGs or pulse oximeter.
- Provide adequate hydration and nutrition.
- Administer mucolytics and encourage effective coughing and deep breathing. Provide chest physiotherapy.
- Change patient's position frequently to enhance clearance of secretions and improve ventilation. Place in semi-Fowler position.
- Give antibacterials to which the known causative bacteria are sensitive. Consider:
  - Uncomplicated CAP: clarithromycin (Biaxin), azithromycin (Zithromax), erythromycin, doxycycline (Vibramycin).
  - Complicated CAP: clarithromycin (Biaxin), azithromycin (Zithromax), erythromycin, moxifloxacin (Avelox), levofloxacin (Levaquin), gemifloxacin (Factive), gatifloxacin (Tequin).

Pneumothorax

Pneumothorax is defined as air entering the pleural space and interrupting the negative pressure, which results in partial or total lung collapse.
Types of pneumothorax include:

- **Spontaneous pneumothorax:** Rupture of subpleural bleb with unknown cause that may be related to smoking and connective tissue disorder. Patients with chronic lung disease (COPD) have a higher incidence.
- **Traumatic pneumothorax:** Caused by blunt chest trauma, penetrating injury, pulmonary contusion → rib fracture or puncture directly to the lung → penetrates parietal and visceral pleura → punctures the lung parenchyma → lung air pressure from positive to negative pressure

environment (inside the lung) → pneumothorax. If pneumothorax remains confined → ↑ air in pleural space on inspiration → air cannot exit on expiration → pressure ↑.

- **Tension pneumothorax:** Due to increased pressure in the pleural space causing the lung to collapse. The increase in pressure may impair circulation by compressing the heart and vena cava.

Pneumothorax can also be categorized by size:

- Small pneumothorax (<15%)
- Moderate pneumothorax (15%–60%)
- Large pneumothorax (>60%)

Clinical Presentation
Pneumothorax presents with:

- Shortness of breath, dyspnea.
- Sharp pleuritic chest pain that increases with deep inspiration and cough on the ipsilateral side. Pain may radiate to the shoulder, neck, or epigastrium.
- Decreased breath sounds, hyperresonance to percussion, absent tactile fremitus on the affected side.
- Hypoxemia, decreased SpO_2 or SaO_2.
- Tachycardia, hypotension.
- Subcutaneous emphysema → swelling in affected area with crepitus upon auscultation.

Can develop into tension pneumothorax → severe respiratory distress, cyanosis, absent breath sounds on the affected side, sinus tachycardia >140 bpm → tracheal deviation → midline shift, hypotension, changes in mental status

Diagnostic Tests
- CXR
- CT scan
- ECG

Management
- Assess vital signs, skin color, breathing pattern, pain level, and oxygenation.
- Keep patient upright.
- Administer O_2 as needed by nasal cannula or mask, and monitor O_2 saturation.

- Use needle aspiration to remove accumulating air.
- Insert chest tube.
- In the case of a small pneumothorax (no symptoms and uncomplicated), observe and monitor the patient for pneumothorax resolution at 1.25% every day.

Pulmonary Edema

Pulmonary edema is defined as abnormal accumulation of fluid in the alveoli, lung tissues, or airway.

Pathophysiology

Inadequate LV function → blood backs up into the pulmonary venous system → ↑ pressure in the pulmonary vasculature → forces intravascular fluid into alveoli and interstitial spaces of lungs → impaired gas exchange → respiratory distress.

Risk factors include:

- Excess fluid in pulmonary capillaries (e.g., HF)
- Cocaine-induced pulmonary vasoconstriction
- Leakage of pulmonary capillary membrane (e.g., ARDS, pneumonia)

Clinical Presentation

- Weak peripheral pulses
- Capillary refill >3 seconds
- Peripheral cyanosis
- Tachycardia
- Tachypnea
- Decreased SpO_2 or PaO_2 with dyspnea
- Decreased cardiac output
- Pallor, diaphoresis
- Vasoconstriction
- Arrhythmias
- Respiratory distress: SOB, decreased respiratory rate, crackles at lung base
- Decreased urine output
- Cough
- Pink, foamy, and frothy sputum
- Change in mental status

Diagnostic Tests

- CXR
- ABGs and/or pulse oximetry
- ECG
- Plasma B-type natriuretic peptide (BNP) level
  - Normal level: 34–42 pg/mL (11.0–13.6 pmol/L)
- Serum cardiac markers
- Two-dimensional transthoracic echocardiogram
- Transesophageal echocardiogram

Management

- Maintain sitting position if BP reading permits.
- Start IV and obtain ABGs.
- Administer O_2 of 5–6 L/min by simple face mask or 1–15 L/min by nonrebreather mask with reservoir and keep SpO_2 >90%.
- Increase O_2 concentration if needed. If unable to resolve respiratory distress, intubation or mechanical ventilation is needed. Consider PEEP.
- Monitor patient with cardiac monitor and pulse oximeter.
- If systolic BP >100, administer nitroglycerin.
- Administer diuretic: IV furosemide (Lasix) 0.5–1 mg/kg.
- Administer morphine slowly if BP is stable.
- Treat the underlying cause.

Pulmonary Arterial Hypertension (PAH)

PAH is defined as a mean pulmonary artery pressure (PAP_m) ≥25 mm Hg and a PCWP ≤15 mm Hg as measured by cardiac catheterization, with a resultant increased pulmonary vascular resistance.

Pathophysiology

PAH is seen in preexisting pulmonary or cardiac disease, familial pulmonary or cardiac disease, chronic obstructive pulmonary disease (COPD), obesity, alveolar hypoventilation, smoke inhalation, high altitude, collagen vascular disease, and congenital heart disease.

Hypoxemia → hypertrophy of smooth muscle in pulmonary arteries → ↓ lumen vessel size → vasoconstriction → narrow of artery vessels → resistance to blood flow → right ventricle pumps harder to move blood across the resistance→ ↑ pulmonary vascular resistance→ ↑ right ventricle workload

$\rightarrow$ smooth muscle proliferated $\rightarrow$ vascular obliteration $\rightarrow$ luminal obstruction $\rightarrow$ $\uparrow$ pulmonary artery pressure and PVR $\rightarrow$ right ventricle hypertrophy, right heart dilation, $\downarrow$ RV cardiac function.

Clinical Presentation

- Increased mean right atrial pressure, decreased cardiac index, increased PAP_m
- ECG: Increased P-wave amplitude (lead II), incomplete right bundle-branch block (RBBB), tall right precordial R waves, right axis deviation, and right ventricular strain
- Hypoxemia, central cyanosis
- Labored and painful breathing, crackles, wheezing
- Jugular venous distention (JVD), hepatomegaly
- Atrial gallop, narrow splitting of S2 or increased S2 intensity, ejection click
- Heart palpitations, angina-like chest pain
- LVF: SOB, hypoventilation, tachypnea, coughing, fatigue, syncope, hypotension, decreased urinary output, decreased cardiac output, shock
- RVF: Peripheral edema, tricuspid regurgitation, prominent heave over right ventricle palpated
- Hoarseness if pressure on left recurrent laryngeal nerve

Diagnostic Tests

- Electrocardiogram
- Two-dimensional echocardiogram with Doppler flow
- CXR or CT
- Polysomnography for PAH sleep-disordered breathing
- V/Q scan—Contraindicated in patients with primary pulmonary hypertension
- Pulmonary angiography with right-sided heart catheterization
- Pulmonary function tests
- ABGs, CBC

Management

- Therapy is dependent upon the stage of the disease.
- The aim is to decrease pulmonary pressure, remove excessive fluid, and decrease the risk of clotting.
- Hemodynamic monitoring.
- Oxygen therapy: Cannula, mask, ventilator.

- Stand-by therapeutic phlebotomy if Hct >60%.
- Low-sodium diet and fluid restrictions.
- Vasodilators, digoxin (Lanoxin), anticoagulants, judicious use of diuretics.
- Administer calcium channel blockers (not for patients with cor pulmonale): nifedipine (Procardia), diltiazem (Cardizem), amlodipine (Norvasc); avoid verapamil (negative inotropic effects).
- Administer prostanoids: treprostinil (Remodulin), iloprost.
- Administer endothelin-receptor antagonists: bosentan (Tracleer), sitaxsentan, ambrisentan.
- Administer phosphodiesterase type 5 (PDE5) inhibitors: sildenafil (Viagra).
- Surgury (optional): Atrial septostomy, pulmonary thromboendarterectomy.
- Lung or heart-lung transplant.

Pulmonary Embolism

Pulmonary embolism is defined as an obstruction of the pulmonary artery or its branch (pulmonary vasculature) by a thrombus or thrombi (blood clot) that originates in the venous circulatory system or the right side of the heart.

Pathophysiology

Usually the result of deep vein thrombosis (DVT) in the legs. Also femoral, popliteal, and iliac veins. Other types: air, fat especially due to long bone fractures, amniotic fluid, tumors, bone marrow, septic thrombi, vegetations on heart valves.

Risk factors include:

- Venous stasis
- Surgery (GYN, abdominal, thoracic, orthopedic)
- Pregnancy
- Estrogen therapy (BCP, HRT)
- Obesity
- Advanced age
- Carcinomas
- Immobilization
- Trauma
- Heart failure

- Stroke
- Sepsis

Thrombus obstructs the pulmonary artery or branch → ↓ blood flow to lungs → impaired/absent gas exchange → ventilation /perfusion mismatch (dead space ventilation) → platelets accumulate around thrombus → release of endotoxins → constrict regional blood vessels + bronchioles → ↑ pulmonary vascular resistance → ↑ pulmonary arterial pressure → ↓ right ventricular work to maintain pulmonary blood flow → right ventricular failure → ↓ cardiac output → ↓ systemic blood pressure → shock

Clinical Presentation

Symptoms, which depend on size of the thrombus and areas of the occlusion, may include:

- Dyspnea, tachypnea, crackles, cough
- Chest pain (sudden, pleuritic, sharp), angina pectoris, myocardial infraction (MI)
- Mental confusion, restlessness
- Leg cramps
- Nausea and vomiting
- Hemoptysis, syncope
- Cardiac arrhythmias, palpitations, hypotension, S3 or S4 gallop
- Anxiety, apprehension
- Fever (>37.8°C), diaphoresis, chills
- Acute cor pulmonale
- Hypoxemia with PaO_2 <80 mm Hg and SaO_2 <95%

Diagnostic Tests

- CXR
- ECG (tall, peaked P wave; tachycardia; atrial fibrillation; RBBB)
- ESR, WBC
- ABGs (low PaO_2)
- D-dimer assay
- Venous ultrasonography and impedance plethysmography
- Ventilation-perfusion V/Q scan
- Pulmonary angiography
- Contrast-enhanced spiral chest CT scan
- High-resolution helical CT angiography

Management

- Provide oxygen by cannula, mask, or ventilator.
- Start heparin infusion.
- Administer sodium bicarbonate if acidotic.
- Monitor prothrombin time (PT), partial thromboplastin time (PTT), international normalized ratio (INR).
- Administer pain medication if needed.
- Administer heparin bolus.
- Elevate head of bed; elevate lower extremities if DVT present.
- Assess vital signs and lung sounds frequently.
- Prepare for surgical embolectomy–intracaval filter
- Administer thrombolytic drug therapy: Recombinant tissue plasminogen activator (TPA), reteplase, streptokinase, urokinase, alteplase.
- Administer morphine to manage pain and anxiety.
- Administer inotropic agents if heart failure present.
- Prevention:
  - Enoxaparin (Lovenox) 30–40 mg daily.
  - Dalteparin (Fragmin) 2,500–5,000 units presurgery and postoperatively.
  - Heparin 5,000 units every 8 hours.
  - Leg exercises—dorsiflexion of the feet.
  - Frequent position changes, ambulation.
  - Antiembolism stockings.

Carbon Monoxide (CO) Poisoning

CO poisoning is defined as an abnormal level of CO in the bloodstream. Normal carboxyhemoglobin (COHgb) level for nonsmokers is <2%; for smokers it is 5% but may be as high as 13%.

Carboxyhemoglobin COHgb level >60% → cardiac toxicity, neurotoxicity, systemic acidosis, respiratory arrest, death.

Pathophysiology

Carbon monoxide (CO) affinity for Hgb is 300 times that of O_2. CO binds with Hgb → ↓ O_2 binding sites → more CO binds → carboxyhemoglobin forms → CO changes structure of Hgb molecules → more difficult for O_2 to bind → tissue ischemia and hypoxemia → acute respiratory failure, ARDS, end organ dysfunction and death.

CO as an inflammatory mediator → tissue damage with ↑ capillary leakage and edema → tracheal and bronchial constriction.

CO → ↓ activity of nitric oxide → (1) peripheral vasodilation → ↓ cerebral blood flow and systemic hypotension; (2) formation of free radicals → endothelial damage and oxidative damage to brain; myocardial depression and arrhythmias → ↓ cardiac output → impaired tissue perfusion.

Clinical Presentation
Early signs

- Headache
- Nausea
- Vomiting
- General fatigue
- Difficulty staying focused
- Flu-like symptoms

Later signs

- Chest pain
- Palpitations
- Dysrhythmias
- MI
- Pulmonary edema
- Throbbing headache, weakness, fatigue, dizziness, memory loss, ataxia, confusion, inability to concentrate
- Skin pale to reddish purple (not a reliable sign)
- Blurred vision, retinal hemorrhages
- Tachypnea, dyspnea, respiratory alkalosis
- Nausea, vomiting, lactic acidosis, rhabdomyolysis
- Upper airway obstruction—hoarseness, dry cough, labored breathing, stridor, difficulty swallowing
- Brassy cough with carbonaceous (soot or carbon) sputum
- Wheezing, bronchospasm

Diagnostic Tests
- COHgb and myoglobin concentration, CBC, CK
- ABG (pulse oximetry inaccurate)
- ECG and CXR
- Fiberoptic bronchoscopy and ventilation/perfusion (V/Q) scan

Management

- Monitor COHgb levels until <10%.
- Administer 100% O_2 via rebreather mask or ETT (mechanical ventilation) to increase PaO_2 levels and decrease $PaCO_2$ levels.
- Assess loss of consciousness (LOC) using Glasgow Coma Scale.
- Monitor pH level if lactic acidosis present.
- Monitor cardiac status. Myocardial injury is a common consequence of moderate to severe CO poisoning → higher risk of death.
- Administer hyperbaric O_2 therapy within 2–6 hours after exposure if symptoms are severe or if COHgb levels ≥25% (controversial).

Thoracic Procedures

Thoracic Surgery

Segmental resection is the removal of the bronchus, a portion of the pulmonary artery and vein, and tissue of the involved lung segment.

Lobectomy is the removal of an entire lobe of the lung.

Pneumonectomy is the removal of the entire lung, generally due to lung cancer, bronchiectasis, TB, or lung abscess. Removal of the right lung is more dangerous because of its larger vascular bed.

Management

Pneumonectomy (postoperative; first 24–48 hours)

- Patient should lie on back or operative side only. This prevents leaking of bronchial stump, prevents fluid from draining into operative site, and allows full expansion of remaining lung.
- Perform CXR to check for deviation of trachea from midline → mediastinal shift.

Patient may need chest tube or thoracostomy needle aspiration.

- Assess for signs and symptoms: neck vein distention, ↑ HR, ↑ RR, dyspnea, trachea displaced to one side.
- Note that remaining lung needs 2–4 days to adjust to increased blood flow.
- Monitor fluid and electrolyte balance to prevent fluid overload (e.g., crackles, increased HR, increased BP, dyspnea).

- Provide oxygen therapy. Mechanical ventilation may be needed; monitor level of oxygenation. Administer pulmonary function tests, such as forced expiratory volume (volume of air patient can forcibly exhale after a full inspiration).
- Encourage coughing, deep breathing, and splinting.
- Elevate head of bed 30°–45°.
- Administer analgesia as needed.
- Monitor ECG to detect cardiac arrhythmias.
- Monitor vital signs to detect hypotension.
- Monitor for pulmonary edema and subcutaneous emphysema.

COMPLICATIONS OF PNEUMONECTOMY

- Atelectasis, pneumothorax, empyema, bronchopleural fistula (increased temperature, cough, increased WBC, anorexia, purulent sputum)
- Excessive blood loss, hemorrhage
- Respiratory distress and pulmonary edema
- Cardiac dysrhythmias and hypotension

Chest Tubes

A chest tube is inserted into the pleural space to reestablish negative intrapleural pressure or to remove air, fluid, or blood. It is inserted after cardiac surgery, if needed, and to treat pneumothorax and hemothorax.

A mediastinal tube is inserted into the mediastinal space to provide fluid and blood drainage after cardiac surgery. It is managed the same as a chest tube.

Management
- Perform CXR immediately after insertion and every day thereafter.
- Apply sterile occlusive gauze dressing to the chest tube site.
- Attach chest tube to water seal drainage; use wall suction.
- Monitor vital signs every 15 minutes until stable, then every 4 hours.
- Monitor color and amount of drainage every 2 hours. Notify physician if drainage >100–200 mL/hr.
- Administer O_2 via nasal cannula or mask; monitor oxygenation.
- Reposition patient every 2 hours.
- Make sure all connections are tight.

- Palpate for subcutaneous emphysema around insertion site and chest wall.
- Auscultate breath sounds; assess respirations.
- Observe color and consistency of drainage; mark fluid level of drainage.
- Check water seal level; add sterile water if needed.
- Avoid clamping the chest tube; can lead to tension pneumothorax.
- Never clamp the chest tube to transport the patient.

Signs of air leak may include bubbles in water seal chamber during inspiration, coughing, and large area of subcutaneous emphysema. Locate source of air leak by gently clamping chest tube near insertion site. If bubbling stops → leak is at the insertion site or inside the patient. If bubbling persists → leak in the system → replace chest tube, retape connections or replace drainage system.

Suction control chamber should be set to 20-cm H_2O level. Fluid level regulates amount of suction → low → add sterile water to chamber. Bubbling should be constant but gentle → "slow boil."

Complications:

- Rapid and shallow breathing
- Cyanosis
- Hemorrhage
- Significant changes in vital signs
- Increased subcutaneous emphysema

Chest tube removal (when there is no air leak for 24 hr, drainage <100 mL/day, and CXR shows complete lung expansion):

- Premedicate with analgesics $\frac{1}{2}$ hour prior to removal.
- Use Vaseline gauze on a sterile dressing and hold over chest tube site. Have patient take a deep breath and perform Valsalva maneuver → chest tube is removed while rapidly covering the chest tube insertion site with the gauzed dressing.
- Perform follow-up CXR.

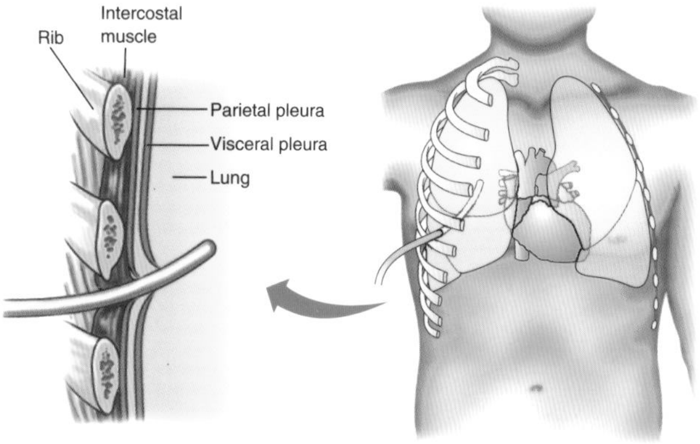

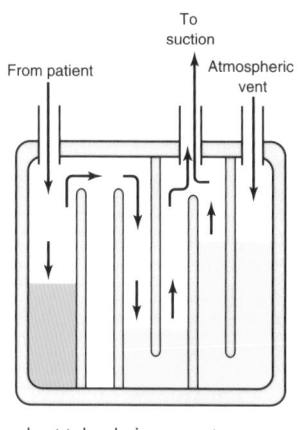

Chest tube placement between ribs and pleural space of lung.

Chamber flow in a chest tube drainage system.

Acute Renal Failure (ARF)

- Chronic kidney disease develops slowly over months to years and necessitates the initiation of dialysis or transplantation. Chronic kidney disease is not a critical care issue. Although it is seen regularly in an ICU setting, it is generally not the reason for admission to the ICU.
- Acute renal failure (ARF) is a clinical syndrome characterized by rapid decline in renal function → progressive azotemia and ↑ creatinine. It is associated with oliguria which can progress over hours or days with ↑ in BUN, creatinine, and K^+ with or without oliguria.

Pathophysiology

The 3 types of acute renal failure include:

- **Prerenal failure:** Caused by conditions such as hemorrhage, myocardial infarction, heart failure, cardiogenic shock, sepsis, and anaphylaxis → impaired blood flow to kidneys → hypoperfusion of kidneys → retention of excessive amount of nitrogenous compounds → intense vasoconstriction → ↓ glomerular filtration rate (GFR). Patient can recover if fluid is replaced.
- **Intrarenal failure:** Caused by burns, crush injuries, infections, glomerulonephritis, lupus erythematosus, diabetes mellitus, malignant HTN, nephroseptic agents → acute tubular necrosis → afferent arteriole vasoconstriction → hypoperfusion of the glomerular apparatus → ↓ GFR → obstruction of tubular lumen by debris and casts, interstitial edema, or release of intrarenal vasoactive substances. A nonrecovery is common.
- **Postrenal failure:** Caused by any obstruction such as bladder tumors, renal calculi, enlarged prostate, or blocked catheter between the kidneys and urethral meatus → ↑ pressure in kidney tubules → ↓ GFR.

Clinical Presentation

ARF presents as:

- Critical illness
- Lethargic
- Persistent nausea and vomiting

- Diarrhea
- Dry skin and mucous membrane from dehydration
- Drowsiness
- Headache
- Muscle twitching
- Seizures

Signs of ARF include:

- Urine <400 mL/24 hours
- ↑ serum urea and creatinine
- Peripheral and systemic edema
- ↓ BP → fluid overload → pulmonary and peripheral edema
- ↓ BP → dehydration/sepsis
- Abnormal, irregular pulse → cardiac arrhythmia
- Kussmaul's respirations → metabolic acidosis
- ↑ temperature → infection
- ↓ level of consciousness (LOC)/seizures
- Electrolyte imbalance (increased serum BUN, creatinine, K^+, Na^+, phosphate; decreased serum calcium)

Diagnostic Tests

- Serum BUN, creatinine, electrolytes, CBC, coagulation studies (PT/PTT), serum osmolality, chemistry panel
- Urinalysis with microscopic examination for protein and casts
- Urine culture and sensitivity
- Urine electrolytes and urine osmolality
- 24-hour urine for creatinine clearance
- Renal ultrasound scanning
- Chest x-ray
- Renal biopsy
- GFR rate
- Kidney-ureters-bladder (KUB) x-ray
- Intravenous pyelogram (IVP)
- CT scan or MRI of kidneys
- Renal arteriogram

Management

- Monitor fluid and electrolytes. Assess for acid-base imbalances.
- Assess respiratory status and monitor oxygenation. Administer O_2 as indicated.
- Institute cardiac monitor and observe for arrhythmias.
- Insert indwelling Foley catheter.
- Restrict fluid intake and measure intake and output strictly. Assess for edema.
- Assess color, clarity, and amount of urine output. Check specific gravity.
- Institute renal diet with adequate protein and low K^+, Na^+, and phosphorus. Protein may be restricted if BUN and creatinine greatly elevated. Treat anorexia, nausea, and vomiting.
- Monitor daily weight.
- Insertion of a large-bore central line.
- Administer medications, including calcium channel blockers, beta blockers, and diuretics such as bumetanide (Bumex) and furosemide (Lasix).
- Administer iron supplement.
- Monitor hemoglobin and hematocrit levels for anemia and O_2-carrying capacity of hemoglobin.
- Administer blood products or erythropoietin products as needed.
- Maintain meticulous skin care to prevent skin breakdown.
- Ensure prevention of secondary infections.
- Assess for gastrointestinal and cutaneous bleeding.
- Assess neurological status for changes in LOC and confusion.
- Administer dialysis (hemodialysis, peritoneal dialysis).
- Provide patient and family support.

Treatment of Renal Disorders

Renal Replacement Therapy

Renal replacement therapy (RRT) is a general term used to describe the various substitution treatments available for severe, acute, and end-stage chronic renal failure (ESCRF), including dialysis (hemodialysis and peritoneal dialysis), hemofiltration, and renal transplant.

Hemodialysis

Hemodialysis is one of several RRTs used in the treatment of renal failure to remove excess fluids and waste products → restores chemical and electrolyte imbalances.

Pathophysiology

Hemodialysis involves passing the client's blood through an artificial semipermeable membrane to perform filtering and excretion functions that the kidney can no longer do effectively.

Procedure

Dialysis works by using passive transfer of toxins by diffusion (movement of molecules from an area of higher concentration to an area of lower concentration). Blood and dialysate (dialyzing solution) containing electrolytes and H_2O (closely resembling plasma) flow in opposite directions through the semipermeable membrane. The patient's blood contains excess H_2O, and excess electrolyte and metabolic waste. During dialysis, the waste products and excess H_2O move from blood → dialysate because of the differences in concentrations. Electrolytes can move in or out of blood or dialysate. This circulating pattern takes place over a preset length of time, generally 3–4 hours.

Components

The components of the hemodialysis system include:

- Dialyzer
- Dialysate
- Vascular access
- Hemodialysis machine

Heparin is used to prevent blood clots from forming in the dialyzer or in the blood tubing. The heparin dose is adjusted to client needs.

Hemodialysis Nursing Care

- Many drugs are dialyzable.
- Vasoactive drugs can cause hypotension → may hold until after dialysis.
- Many antibiotics are given after dialysis and administered on days patients receive dialysis.

Postdialysis Care

- Monitor vital signs every hour x 4 hours, then every 4 hours (hypotension may occur secondary to hypovolemia requiring IV fluids; ↑ temperature may occur after dialysis secondary to blood warming mechanism of the hemodialysis machine).
- Weigh postdialysis.
- Avoid all invasive procedures for 4–6 hours after dialysis if anticoagulation used.

Continuous Renal Replacement Therapy (CRRT)

Continuous renal replacement therapy (CRRT) represents a family of modalities that provide continuous support of severely ill patients in ARF. It is used when hemodialysis is not feasible. CRRT works more slowly than hemodialysis and requires continuous monitoring. It is indicated for patients who are no longer responding to diuretic therapy, are in fluid overload, and/or are hemodynamically unstable.

Procedure

CRRT requires placement of a continuous arteriovenous hemofiltration (CAVH) catheter or continuous venovenous hemofiltration (CVVH) catheter and a mean arterial pressure of 60 mm Hg.

Other types of CRRT include:

- Continuous arteriovenous hemodialysis (CAVHD)
- Continuous venovenous hemodialysis (CVVHD)
- Slow continuous ultrafiltration (SCUF)
- Continuous arteriovenous hemodiafiltration (CAVHDF)
- Continuous venovenous hemodiafiltration (CVVHDF)

Because it is difficult to obtain and maintain arterial access, CVVH or venous access is preferred.

CRRT provides for the removal of fluid, electrolytes, and solutes.

CRRT differs from hemodialysis in the following ways:

- It is continuous rather than intermittent, and large fluid volumes can be removed over days instead of hours.
- Solute removal can occur by convection (no dialysate required) in addition to osmosis and diffusion.
- It causes less hemodynamic instability.

- It requires a trained ICU RN to care for patient but does not require constant monitoring by a specialized hemodialysis nurse.
- It does not require hemodialysis equipment, but a modified blood pump is required.
- It is the ideal treatment for someone who needs fluid and solute control but cannot tolerate rapid fluid removal.
- It can be administered continuously, for as long as 30–40 days. The hemofilter is changed every 24–48 hours.

Nursing Care
- Monitor fluid and electrolyte balance.
- Monitor intake and output every hour.
- Weigh daily.
- Monitor vital signs every hour.
- Assess and provide care of vascular access site every shift.

Renal Transplant

A renal transplant is the surgical placement of a cadaveric kidney or live donor kidney (including all arterial and venous vessels and long piece of ureter) into a patient with end-stage renal disease (ESRD).

Operative Procedure
The surgery takes 4–5 hours. The transplanted kidney is usually placed in the right iliac fossa to allow for easier access to the renal artery, vein, and ureter attachment. The patient's nonfunctioning kidney usually stays in place unless there is a concern about chronic infection in one or both kidneys.

Postoperative Care
- Admit to ICU.
- Monitor vital signs frequently as per ICU policy.
- Monitor hourly urine output for first 48 hours.
- Assess urine color.
- Obtain daily urinalysis, urine electrolytes, urine for acetones, and urine culture and sensitivity.
- Administer immunosuppressive drug therapy (↑ risk of infection).
- Provide Foley catheter care.
- Maintain continuous bladder irrigation as needed.
- Strict intake and output.
- Monitor daily weight.

- Administer diuretics.
- Obtain daily basic metabolic panel (BMP).

Complications

- Rejection (most common and serious complication): A reaction between the antigens in the transplanted kidney and the antibodies in the recipient's blood → tissue destruction → kidney necrosis.
- Thrombosis to the major renal artery, may occur up to 2–3 days postop → may be indicated by sudden ↓ in urine output → emergent surgery is required to prevent ischemia to the kidney.
- Renal artery stenosis → HTN is the manifestation of this complication → a bruit over the graft site or ↓ in renal function may be other indicators → may be repaired surgically or by balloon angioplasty.
- Vascular leakage or thrombosis → requires emergent nephrectomy surgery.
- Wound complications: Hematomas, abscesses → ↑ risk of infection → exertion on new kidney. Infection is major cause of death in transplant recipient. These patients are on immunosuppressive therapy → signs and symptoms of infection may not manifest in its usual way. Watch for low-grade fevers, mental status changes, and vague complaints of discomfort.

Nephrectomy

Radical nephrectomy is the removal of the kidney, the ipsilateral adrenal gland, surrounding tissue, and, at times, surrounding lymph nodes. Due to the increased risk of reoccurrence in the ureteral stump, a ureterectomy may be performed as well.

Pathophysiology

Primary indication is for treatment of renal cell carcinoma (adenocarcinoma of the kidney), in which the healthy tissue of the kidney is destroyed and replaced by cancer cells.

Secondary indication is for treatment of renal trauma → penetrating wounds or blunt injuries to back, flank, or abdomen injuring the kidney; injury or laceration to the renal artery → hemorrhage.

Clinical Presentation

- Flank pain (dull, aching)
- Gross hematuria

- Palpable renal mass
- Abdominal discomfort (present in 5%–10% of cases)
- Hematuria (late sign)
- Muscle wasting, weakness, poor nutritional status, weight loss (late signs)

Diagnostic Tests
- Urinalysis (may show RBCs)
- Complete blood count
- Complete metabolic panel (CMP)
- Erythrocyte sedimentation rate (ESR or sed rate)
- Human chorionic gonadotropin (hCG) level
- Cortisol level
- Adrenocorticotropic hormone level
- Renin level
- Parathyroid hormone level
- Surgical exploration
- IV urogram
- Nephrogram
- Sonogram
- CT of abdomen/pelvis with contrast
- MRI

Postop Management
- Monitor vital signs frequently.
- Provide pain management.
- Encourage patient to cough and deep breathe, and to use incentive spirometer every hour.
- Encourage early mobilization.
- Monitor intake and output strictly.
- Assess for bleeding.
- Administer IV fluids.
- May require blood transfusion.
- Obtain CBC every 6 hours x 24 hours, then every 12 hours for 24 hours early postop.
- Monitor daily weight.
- Monitor for adrenal insufficiency.
- If drain in place, monitor and record color and amount of drainage.

Cystectomy

A radical cystectomy is the removal of the bladder, prostate, and seminal vesicles in men; and the bladder, ureters, cervix, urethra, and ovaries in women. The ureters are diverted into collection reservoirs → urinary diversion (ileal conduit, continent pouch, bladder reconstruction [neobladder], ureterosigmoidostomy).

Pathophysiology
Primary indication is for treatment of carcinoma of the bladder (transitional cell, squamous cell, or adenocarcinoma). Once the cancer spreads beyond the transitional cell layer, the risk of metastasis ↑ greatly.

Secondary indication is as part of pelvic exoneration for sarcomas or tumors of the GI tract or GYN system.

Clinical Presentation
■ Gross painless hematuria (chronic or intermittent)
■ Bladder irritability with dysuria, urgency, and frequency
■ Urine cytology positive for neoplastic or atypical cells
■ Urine tests positive for bladder tumor antigens

Diagnostic Tests
■ Urine cytology
■ Urine for bladder tumor antigens
■ IV pyelogram
■ Ultrasound of bladder, kidneys, and ureters
■ CT of abdomen and pelvis
■ MRI of abdomen and pelvis
■ Cystoscopy and biopsy (confirmation of bladder carcinoma)

Postop Management
■ Monitor vital signs frequently, as per hospital policy immediately postoperatively.
■ Encourage patient to cough and deep breathe, and to use incentive spirometer every hour.
■ Monitor and record amount of bleeding from incision and in urine.
■ Monitor and record intake and output.
■ If patient has a cutaneous urinary diversion, assess stoma for warmth and color every 8 hours in early postop period (ostomy appliance will collect urine).

- Collaborate with enteral stoma nurse regarding stoma, skin, and urinary drainage.
- If Penrose drain or plastic catheters in place, monitor and record drainage.
- Monitor hemoglobin and hematocrit levels.
- Provide pain management.
- Encourage early ambulation.
- Provide patient and family support.

Increased Intracranial Pressure

Increased ICP is an increase in pressure on the brain within the cranium or skull caused by an increase in cerebrospinal fluid pressure. Normal ICP is 1–15 mm Hg.

Cerebral perfusion pressure is a function of the mean arterial pressure and intracranial pressure. If the CPP drops below 80 mm Hg, ischemia may occur.

CPP should be maintained at 70–80 mm Hg and the ICP at <15 mm Hg.
Cerebral perfusion pressure (CPP) = mean arterial pressure (MAP) – ICP.
MAP = systolic blood pressure + 2 (diastolic blood pressure) ÷ 3.

Pathophysiology

- Risk factor → ↑ intracranial volume of cerebrospinal fluid (CSF) → ↑ ICP → ↓ cerebral perfusion, ↑ brain swelling → a shift in brain tissue through the dura → herniation → death. Increased ICP also leads to brain tissue ischemia/infarction and brain death.
- Herniation results in a downward shifting of brain tissue from an area of high pressure to low pressure, usually into the brainstem → coma and death.

Clinical Presentation

- Slow, bounding pulse and irregular respirations
- Headache and changes in level of consciousness, slow speech, restlessness, confusion, ↑ drowsiness
- Stupor, coma, decortication, decerebration, and flaccidity
- Fixed and dilated pupils
- Respiratory impairment (Cheyne-Stokes), irregular or absence of breathing → death
- Cushing's response/reflex: ↓↓ cerebral blood flow → cerebral ischemia → ↑ arterial pressure and ↑ systolic BP, bradypnea, widening pulse pressure and reflex bradycardia (late sign).

Decerebrate Position

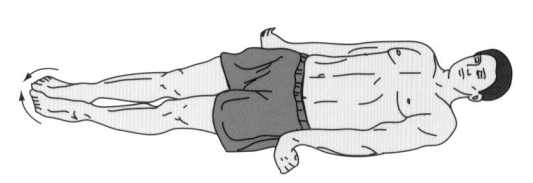

Decorticate Position

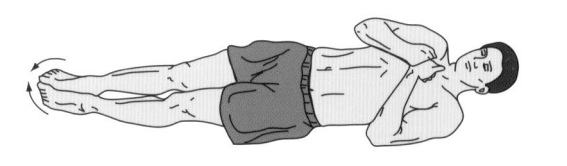

Complications

- Brainstem herniation, brain anoxia, death
- Diabetes insipidus
- Syndrome of inappropriate antidiuretic hormone (SIADH)

Diagnostic Tests

- Serum electrolytes and serum osmolarity
- Cerebral angiography, CT scan, MRI, PET to rule out physiological cause
- Transcranial Doppler studies
- Avoid lumbar puncture, can lead to brain herniation
- ICP monitoring devices: Ventricular drainage, intracranial bolts, intra-parenchymal fiber-optic catheter

Management

- Treatment is based on trends and sustained elevations of ICP and low CPP.

- Administer osmotic diuretic (mannitol [Osmitrol] 0.25–1 g/kg). Restrict fluids if necessary.
- Administer diuretics such as furosemide (Lasix).
- Administer IV hypertonic saline (>0.9% NaCl).
- Institute mechanical ventilation according to arterial blood gases (ABGs).
- Administer IV sedation cautiously.
- Assess neurological and mental status by Glasgow Coma Scale, including reflexes, pupils, motor and sensory function, and cranial nerve function (extraocular movements, peripheral facial droop, tongue deviation, gag reflex, corneal reflex, cough reflex, doll's eyes).
- Assess for meningeal signs (headache, nuchal [neck] rigidity, photophobia).
- Assess response to verbal and painful stimuli.
- Institute seizure precautions; administer anticonvulsants as necessary.
- Monitor vital signs, CPP, and ICP, and control fever; hypothermia use is controversial.
- Keep head in midline position (head of bed [HOB] 30°–60°).
- Avoid extreme rotation of neck and neck flexion.
- Avoid extreme hip flexion.
- Maintain patent airway, suction cautiously (can ↑ ICP), oxygenate, and avoid positive end-expiratory pressure (PEEP).
- Monitor ABGs and oxygenation.
- Maintain cardiac output using inotropes such as dobutamine (Dobutrex) and norepinephrine (Levophed).
- Administer high doses of barbiturates to ↓ ICP (pentobarbital [Nembutal], thiopental [Pentothal], and propofol [Diprivan] to ↓ metabolic demands).
- Administer anticonvulsants.
- Induce therapeutic hypothermia.
- Provide DVT and peptic ulcer prophylaxis.
- The following can ↑ intracranial pressure and should be avoided: hypercapnia, hypoxemia, Valsalva maneuver, isometric muscle contractions, REM sleep, and noxious stimuli.

Glasgow Coma Scale				
Response	**Patient Response**	**Score**	**Patient A**	**Patient B**
Eye opening response	Spontaneous	4		
	To voice	3		
	To pain	2		
	None	1		
Best verbal response	Oriented	5		
	Confused	4		
	Inappropriate words	3		
	Incomprehensible sounds	2		
	None	1		
Best motor response	Obeys command	6		
	Localizes pain	5		
	Withdraws	4		
	Flexion	3		
	Extension	2		
	None	1		
Total		3–15		

A score of 8 or less indicates severe head injury.

Reprinted from The Lancet, Vol. 304, Teasdale G and Jennett B, Assessment of Coma and Impaired Consciousness: A Practical Scale, Page 4, Copyright (1994), with permission from Elsevier.

ICP Monitoring

Devices placed inside the head that sense the pressure inside the brain cavity and send measurement to a recording device include:

- Intraventricular catheter (ventriculostomy), which allows CSF to drain and allows for intraventricular administration of medications
- Subarachnoid bolt or screw
- Epidural or subdural catheter or sensor

Calibrate transducer 1 inch above ear with patient in supine position.

Risks

- Infection and bleeding
- Damage to the brain tissue → neurological effects
- Inability to accurately place catheter

Troubleshooting ICP Monitoring Problems

- Check all connections; reposition catheter.
- Check for air in the system.
- Check monitor cable.
- Calibrate or reposition transducer.

ICP Catheter Waveforms

- A (plateau) waves → cerebral ischemia
- B waves → intracranial hypertension (HTN) and change in vascular volume
- C waves → variations in systemic arterial pressure and respirations

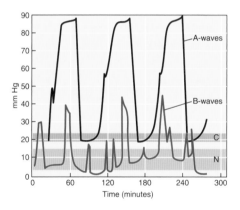

Brain Monitoring

Cerebral or jugular venous oxygen saturation ($SjvO_2$) (virtually all blood from the brain drains into internal jugular veins):

- 60%–80% is normal
- <50% indicates cerebral hypoxia
- Brain tissue O_2 monitoring (partial pressure of brain tissue O_2 [$PbtO_2$] using LICOX catheter): >25 mm Hg is normal; <20 mm Hg needs to be treated
- Brain temperature monitoring: $0.5°–1.0°$ C > core body temperature is normal
- Bispectral index (BIS): EEG of critically ill patients with a decreased level of consciousness is continually analyzed

Traumatic Brain Injury

Traumatic brain injury refers to trauma to the scalp and skull that may or may not include injury to the brain. There are several types of acute head injuries:

- Closed head injury: The skull is not broken
- Penetrating head injury: Object pierces the skull and breaches the dura mater
- May also be diffuse or focal

Pathophysiology

Trauma → intracranial hemorrhage and hematoma → brain swelling → ↑ intracranial volume and ↑ ICP → displacement or herniation of the brain. Pressure on cerebral blood vessels → ↓ blood flow to brain → ↓ O_2 to brain → cerebral hypoxia → cerebral ischemia, infarction, and irreversible brain damage → brain death.

Clinical Presentation

- Persistent, localized pain; headache
- Loss of consciousness, confusion, drowsiness, personality change, restlessness

- Sudden onset of neurological deficits
- Bruising over mastoid (Battle's sign)
- Nausea and vomiting
- CSF otorrhea (ears) or rhinorrhea (nose)
- Halo sign: Blood stain surrounded by a yellowish stain on bed linens or head dressing that may indicate CSF leak
- Abnormal pupillary response
- Altered or absent gag reflex
- Absent corneal reflex
- Change in vital signs: altered respiratory pattern, widened pulse pressure, bradycardia, or tachycardia
- Seizures

Complicating Factors

- Skull fracture, scalp lacerations
- Cerebral contusion, concussion
- Subarachnoid hemorrhage
- Subdural, extra/epidural hematoma
- Cerebral edema
- ↑ ICP ↓ cerebral perfusion
- Seizures
- Impaired oxygenation/ventilation
- Herniation, coma, or death

Diagnostic Tests

- Check for cerebrospinal fluid leak
- X-ray, CT of the head, MRI, or PET to assess hematoma, swelling, and injury
- Cerebral angiography
- CBC, chemistry panel, and blood coagulation studies
- Urinalysis for specific gravity

Management

- Stabilize cardiac and respiratory function to ensure adequate cerebral perfusion. Maintain optimum ABGs or O_2 saturation. Assess oxygenation and respiratory status.

- Assess and monitor neurological status and ICP; calculate CPP to maintain >70 mm Hg.
- Perform frequent neurological checks, including Glasgow Coma Scale. See pg. 124.
- Provide light sedation as necessary to ↓ agitation. Administer analgesics for pain. Induce barbiturate coma if necessary.
- Administer hypertonic saline and osmotic diuretics as needed.
- Monitor and control for elevations in ICP.
- Induce therapeutic hypothermia.
- Prepare patient for craniotomy to lessen the pressure in the brain if necessary.
- Assess for vision and hearing impairment and sensory function.
- Assess for hypothermia and hyperthermia. Control fever.
- Institute seizure precautions. Minimize stimuli and excessive suctioning.
- Monitor ECG for cardiac arrhythmias. Institute deep vein thrombosis (DVT) precautions.
- Assess fluid and electrolyte balance. Control hemorrhage and hypovolemia.
- Administer stool softeners to prevent Valsalva maneuver.
- Keep head and neck in neutral alignment; no twisting or flexing of neck.
- Keep head of bed elevated.
- Maintain adequate nutrition orally or enterally. Assess and maintain skin integrity.
- Provide DVT and peptic ulcer prophylaxis.

Subarachnoid Hemorrhage or Hemorrhagic Stroke

SAH is bleeding into the subarachnoid space between the arachnoid membrane and the pia mater of the brain primarily. SAH is a medical emergency.

Pathophysiology

- SAH is caused by cerebral aneurysm (usually in the area of circle of Willis), cerebral/head trauma, HTN, or arteriovenous malformation.
- Blood rapidly passes into the subarachnoid space and then spreads over the brain and to the spinal cord leading to ↑ ICP → coma → death.

Clinical Presentation

- Sudden, severe "thunderclap" headache developing over seconds to minutes
- ↓ level of consciousness (LOC); confusion and agitation
- Nuchal rigidity (stiff neck)
- Nausea and vomiting
- Photophobia, diplopia, visual loss, blurred vision, and oculomotor nerve abnormalities (affected eye looking downward and outward, pupil widened and less responsive to light)
- Paralysis; positive Brudzinski's sign and Kernig's sign
- Tinnitus, dizziness, vertigo, and hemiparesis
- Fatigue, fever, and HTN
- Cardiac arrhythmias (can progress to cardiac arrest)

Complications

- Increased ICP
- Coma and brainstem herniation
- Rebleeding
- Cerebral vasospasm
- Hyponatremia due to SIADH or cerebral salt-wasting syndrome
- Cardiac arrhythmias and myocardial damage
- Acute hydrocephalus
- Pneumonia, pulmonary embolus, and respiratory failure
- Neurogenic cardiac stunning (reduction of function of heart contraction) and pulmonary edema

Diagnostic Tests

- CT scan of brain or MRI of brain
- Transcranial Doppler studies
- ECG (changes in ST segment and T wave, prominent U wave)
- Lumbar puncture if CT inconclusive and no ↑ ICP present
- CSF is clear and colorless, with no organisms present; it will test positive for protein and glucose
- Cerebral angiography

NEURO

Management

- Neurological assessment: LOC, papillary reaction, motor and sensory function, cranial nerve deficits, and speech and visual disturbances.
- Assess for headache and nuchal rigidity.
- Provide intubation and mechanical ventilation as needed; assess ABGs.
- Assess BP, HR, RR, and Glasgow Coma Scale frequently.
- Control BP via antihypertensives. Monitor and control ICP.
- Institute aneurysm precautions: Bed rest; dark, quiet room with minimal stimulation and nonstressful environment; pain control; ↑ HOB 15°–30°; stool softeners (avoid enemas). Restrict visitors.
- Avoid Valsalva maneuver, straining, forceful sneezing, and acute flexion of head and neck. Eliminate caffeine from diet.
- Administer analgesia for pain control; use nonsedating agents. Control anxiety.
- Give nimodipine (Nimotop) for cerebral vasodilation. Therapy should start within 96 hours of subarachnoid hemorrhage.
- Provide DVT and peptic ulcer prophylaxis.

Triple-H Therapy to Prevent Vasospasms

- Hypovolemia treated with colloids and crystalloids to keep central venous pressure (CVP) 10–12 mm Hg and pulmonary capillary wedge pressure (PCWP) 15–18 mm Hg
- Hemodilution to keep hematocrit level at 33%–38%
- Hypertensive therapy to keep systolic BP 110–160 mm Hg

Prepare patient for surgery:

- Surgical aneurysm repair: Surgical clipping
- Endovascular treatment: Occlusion of parent artery
- Endovascular (aneurysm) coiling: Obstruction of aneurysm site with coil

Cerebral Vascular Accident–Ischemic Stroke

CVA is a sudden disruption of blood flow to a part of the brain. It may be hemorrhagic (see subarachnoid hemorrhage) or ischemic and may result in brain tissue damage and neurological deficits. CVA is also called brain attack.

Pathophysiology

- Causes of CVA include thrombosis, embolism, systemic hypoperfusion, and hemorrhage. Cocaine use doubles the risk of CVA.
- In CVA there is a disruption of blood flow to the brain → ↓ O_2 and glucose to the brain → ischemic cascade → neurons unable to maintain aerobic respiration → switch to anaerobic respiration → build-up of lactic acid → change in blood pH → influx of intracellular calcium and increase in glutamate → destroys cell membrane → cell membrane and proteins break down, forming free radicals → cell injury and death → neurological dysfunction.
- Low cerebral blood flow → ↓ O_2 to the brain → ↑ extraction of O_2 by the brain.
- Ischemia penumbra (zone of ischemic area) forms around an infarct in stroke lesions. This penumbra may be reversible.

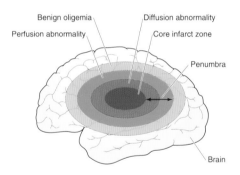

Clinical Presentation

- Sudden neurological deficits such as muscle weakness (hemiplegia) of face, arm, or leg (especially if confined to one side of body); confusion or trouble speaking or understanding speech; trouble seeing

in one or both eyes; trouble walking; dizziness; loss of balance or coordination; and severe headache with no known cause
- Other neurological assessments: Ptosis (drooping of eyelids), weakness of ocular muscles, ↓ gag and swallow reflex, slow papillary reactivity to light, visual field defects, memory defects, confusion, and hypersexual gestures
- Numbness; ↓ sensory or vibratory sensation; altered sense of small, taste, hearing; ↓ sensation and muscle weakness to face (facial paresis); nystagmus; and dysphagia
- Altered breathing and heart rate
- Inability to turn head to one side (weak sternocleidomastoid muscle)
- Inability to protrude tongue and/or move from side to side
- Aphasia (difficulty to speak or understand language)
- Apraxia (altered voluntary movements)
- Vertigo and disequilibrium, with difficulty walking, altered movement coordination, and arm drift
- Urinary and fecal incontinence

Complications

- Physical: Pressure sores, incontinence, pneumonia, seizures, coma, and death
- Emotional: Anxiety, panic attacks, flat affect, depression, withdrawal, sleep disturbances, lethargy, irritability, and emotional lability

Diagnostic Tests

- CBC, serum chemistry, coagulation studies, fibrinogen test
- Drug screen and ETOH level if indicated
- CT scan without contrast or MRI
- Carotid Doppler ultrasound (carotid stenosis)
- Transcranial Doppler flow studies
- ECG, transthoracic of transesophageal echocardiogram, Holter monitor (arrhythmias)
- EEG, especially if seizure activity is present
- ABGs if hypoxic
- Cerebral angiography

Management

- Administer recombinant tissue plasminogen activator (rtPA) within 3 hours of onset of symptoms (contraindicated if abnormal lab values, HTN, or recent surgery). Risk of intracranial bleeding. rtPA may also be administered intra-arterially by the interventional radiologist via the femoral artery within 6 hours of symptoms.
- Administer aspirin (50–325 mg daily), clopidogrel (75 mg daily), or dipyridamole extended release (25/200 mg twice daily) if no rtPA.
- Assess for bleeding related to anticoagulant therapy.
- Induce hypothermia within 12 hours of stroke symptoms by infusing cold saline intravenously into the body until core temperature is 92°F or 33°C.
- Assess and monitor neurological and respiratory function; administer O_2 if necessary. Keep $PaCO_2$ at 30–35 mm Hg and/or SpO_2 at >95%. Avoid hypoxia. Intubate if needed according to ABGs.
- Monitor and manage ↑ ICP and cerebral edema. Give mannitol, furosemide (Lasix), or 3% saline solution. Use nondextrose IV solutions.
- Monitor BP. Management of HTN may be deferred unless end-organ damage, MAP >130 mm Hg, SBP >220 mm Hg, or DBP >120 mm Hg.
- Administer sodium nitroprusside (Nipride) or labetalol (Normodyne, Trandate) IV.
- Ensure continuous cardiac monitoring of arrhythmias.
- Provide DVT and peptic ulcer disease prophylaxis.
- Maintain glycemic control (blood glucose at 80–110 mg/dL) with IV insulin.
- Provide ECG monitoring to prevent bradycardia → ↓ CO and ↓ CPP.
- Treat and control fever.
- Avoid use of Foley catheter if possible. Monitor intake and output closely.
- Institute seizure precautions and administer anticonvulsants if necessary.
- Provide enteral or PEG tube feedings, following aspiration precautions. Elevate HOB 30°.
- Provide DVT and peptic ulcer prophylaxis.

Surgical Management

■ Carotid endarterectomy or carotid artery angioplasty and stenting
■ Mechanical thrombectomy to remove offending thrombus

Spinal Cord Injury

SCI may be classified as complete (loss of conscious sensory and motor function below the level of spinal cord injury due to transaction of the spinal cord) or incomplete (preservation of some sensory and motor function below the level of spinal cord injury due to partial spinal cord transaction). The most common sites of SCI are C4–C7, T12, and L1.

Causes of SCI include:

■ Blunt force trauma
■ Penetrating force trauma
■ Ankylosing spondylitis
■ Rheumatoid arthritis
■ Spinal abscesses and tumors, especially lymphoma and multiple myeloma

Pathophysiology

■ ↓ blood flow to gray matter of spinal cord with 8-hour delay of ↓ blood flow to white matter → thrombi form furthering ↓ blood flow to spinal cord.
■ ↑ interstitial pressure related to edema → ↓ blood flow to spinal cord.
■ Inflammatory process → edema of injured area → ↓ blood flow to spinal cord. Edema moves up and down the spinal cord rather than laterally.
■ Release of norepinephrine, histamine, and prostaglandins → vasoconstriction → ↓ cellular perfusion.
■ ↑ extracellular fluid concentrations of Na^+ and K^+ → ↑ osmotic pressure in area of injury → edema.
■ Ischemia, hypoxia, and edema → tissue necrosis and cell membrane damage → destruction of myelin and axons → neuronal death.

Clinical Presentation

- Spinal shock initially: Flaccid paralysis with $\downarrow$ or absent reflex activity
- Partial or total loss of motor function below the level of SCI (includes voluntary movement and movement against gravity or resistance)
- Partial or total loss of sensory function below the level of SCI (includes touch, temperature, pain, proprioception [e.g., position])
- $\uparrow$ HR initially $\rightarrow$ bradycardia; $\uparrow$ BP initially $\rightarrow$ $\downarrow$ BP
- Acute pain in back or neck that may radiate along nerve
- Abnormal deep tendon reflex and perianal reflex activity
- Loss of sweating and vagomotor tone
- Loss of sensory, motor, and deep tendon reflexes below the level of injury
- Retention of lung secretions, $\downarrow$ vital capacity, $\uparrow$ $PaCO_2$, $\downarrow$ O_2 $\rightarrow$ respiratory failure and pulmonary edema
- Bladder and bowel incontinence with urine retention and bladder distention
- Paralytic ileus causing constipation and/or bowel impaction
- Loss of temperature control $\rightarrow$ hyperthermia
- Sweating above level of lesion
- Priapism in males

Diagnostic Tests

- Lateral, anterior-posterior (cervical, thoracic, lumbar, sacral), and odontoid films
- CT scan, MRI
- Myelography

Management

- Assess motor and sensory function, including deep tendon reflexes.
- Assess neurological status, including LOC and papillary action.
- Assess for closed head injury.
- Maintain spinal and proper body alignment.
- Assess respiratory status. Monitor ABGs or pulse oximetry. Administer O_2 by nasal cannula or mask. Provide mechanical ventilation as determined by ABGs.

NEURO

- Suction cautiously → stimulate vagus nerve → bradycardia → cardiac arrest.
- Monitor ECG for cardiac dysrhythmias, especially bradycardia (may need pacemaker). Monitor BP for hypotension.
- Provide intermittent bladder catheterization or temporary Foley catheter.
- Provide DVT and peptic ulcer prophylaxis.
- Insert nasogastric tube initially to prevent vomiting and aspiration.
- Start TPN or enteral feedings.
- Follow skin care protocol to prevent decubitus ulcers.
- Avoid and treat bladder spasms.
- Avoid bowel impaction by administering stool softeners and establish bowel control.
- Prevent autonomic dysreflexia.
- Provide IV fluids cautiously, because they can precipitate heart failure due to poor heart rate response to ↓ circulating blood volume. Administer methylprednisolone Na succinate within 8 hours of injury (30 mg/kg IV over 15 minutes; infusion of 5.4 mg/kg/hr for 24–48 hours).
- Administer vasodilators: nifedipine (Procardia), phenoxybenzamine (Dibenzyline), or nitroprusside (Nipride).
- Prevent sepsis and infections (respiratory, urinary tract, and wound).
- Provide emotional support for patient and family.
- Prepare patient for surgical management to reduce spinal fracture or dislocation and decompression of the spinal cord:
  - Skeletal fracture reduction and traction with skeletal tongs or calipers, skeletal traction device, and halo device.

Autonomic Dysreflexia

A stimulus causes ↑ sympathetic nervous system response below the level of SCI and systemic vasoconstriction → bradycardia, HTN, facial and neck flushing (reddening above the level of SCI) associated with pale, cold skin on the trunk and extremities (below the SCI), sweating, anxiety, pounding headache, nasal congestion, "goose bumps," blurred vision, difficulty breathing, increased spasticity, and chest pain. It may lead to CVA, renal failure, atrial fibrillation, seizures, and acute pulmonary edema.

Autonomic dysreflexia is also known as hyperreflexia. It occurs in people with SCI at or above the level of T6 (or rarely as low as T8).

Causes

- Bladder distention or spasm (most common cause); urinary tract infection
- Bowel impaction
- Stimulation of anal reflex (stimulation of skin around the anus produces contraction of the anal sphincter)
- Labor in women
- Temperature change
- Acute pain
- Decubitus ulcer
- Tight, constrictive clothes
- Ingrown toenails

Management

- Place patient in sitting position and monitor vital signs every 5 minutes.
- Loosen constrictive clothing or devices.
- If no indwelling catheter, palpate bladder for distention → insert Foley catheter.
- If indwelling catheter, check for kinks and obstruction and irrigate if necessary.
- Check for fecal impaction and administer laxative as needed. Use 2% lidocaine jelly 10–15 minutes before removing impaction.
- Assess skin for pressure or irritation.
- If SBP >150 mm Hg, administer an antihypertensive such as hydralazine (Apresoline).
    - The sweating will become less profuse or stop.
    - There will usually be an immediate lowering of the BP, although it may take about 1 hour for BP to decrease if BP is very high.

Neurogenic Shock

Neurogenic shock is caused by vasoconstriction and venous pooling (veins dilated and filled with blood) → ↓ BP, ↓ systemic vascular resistance, ↓ HR, ↓ CO, ↓ respiration rate, skin warm with pink mucous membranes → ↓ blood flow to vital organs → organ damage and ischemia. Treatment involves the administration of vasopressors.

Myasthenia Gravis

MG is a neuromuscular autoimmune disease causing muscle weakness and fatigability of skeletal muscles.

Pathophysiology

Circulating antibodies block acetylcholine receptors at the postsynaptic neuromuscular junction → inhibits acetylcholine → inhibits depolarization of muscles → ↓ nerve impulse transmission → diminishes muscle contraction, including diaphragmatic muscle → ↓ vital capacity and respiratory failure.

Causes include thymic hyperplasia and tumor of the thymus gland.

Clinical Presentation

- Muscle weakness that increases during activity and improves after rest; eye muscle weakness; possible ptosis, diplopia, and inability to maintain upward gaze
- Weakness of limb, axial, bulbar, and/or respiratory muscles, especially those related to chewing, talking, swallowing (dysphagia), breathing, and neck and limb movements; inability to close mouth and inability to raise chin off chest
- Slurred speech, neck muscle weakness with head bobbing
- Diaphragmatic and intercostal weakness → dyspnea, difficulty coughing
- Crises that may be triggered by fever, infection, trauma, extreme temperatures, adverse reaction to medication or emotional stress → respiratory distress, dysphagia, dysarthria (difficulty speaking), eyelid

ptosis, diplopia, prominent muscle weakness, neurologic changes, absence of sweating, hyperthermia → respiratory failure

Diagnostic Tests

- Muscle fatigability test
- Antibodies against acetylcholine receptor (AChR Ab) ≤0.03 nmol/L or negative
- Edrophonium chloride (Tensilon) test: Administration of 1–2 mg IV over 15–20 seconds; resolution of facial muscle weakness and ptosis and improved muscle strength should be seen in 30 seconds; if no response in 1 minute, may repeat dose; have atropine, ECG monitoring, and advanced life-saving equipment available
- Ice pack test: Placing ice over an eyelid if ptosis is present; clear resolution of the ptosis is a positive test result; ptosis occurs in approximately 80% of patients with ocular myasthenia
- Single-fiber electromyography and repetitive nerve stimulation
- Blood test to identify antibodies against the acetylcholine receptor (AChR Abs)
- Thyroid function and pulmonary function tests
- CT scan or MRI to detect thymomas

Management

- Assess and monitor respiratory status and oxygenation (pulmonary function tests, ABGs).
- Provide mechanical ventilation if paralysis of respiratory muscles is present.
- Monitor risk for aspiration and pneumonia. Initiate enteral feedings if dysphagic.
- Avoid sedatives and tranquilizers.
- Initiate plasmapheresis to treat exacerbations.
- Administer IV immunoglobulin (IVIG).
- Administer immunosuppressants such as:
  - Prednisone
  - Cyclosporine
  - Mycophenolate mofetil

NEURO

- ■ Azathioprine
- ■ Corticosteroids
■ Administer cholinesterase inhibitors: neostigmine (Prostigmin), pyridostigmine (Mestinon).
■ Provide DVT and peptic ulcer prophylaxis.
■ Prepare patient for surgical thymectomy.

Guillain-Barré Syndrome

GBS is an autoimmune acute inflammatory disease causing demyelination of the lower motor neurons of the peripheral nervous system.

Pathophysiology

■ Immune-mediated response → destruction of myelin sheath → interferes with nerve signal transmission → slowing of nerve signals → weakness of limbs → ascending paralysis → total paralysis.
■ Paralysis of the diaphragm → respiratory failure.
■ If mild, remyelination can occur.

Clinical Presentation

■ Infection of the respiratory or GI tract 10–14 days before onset of neurological symptoms
■ Flaccidity of muscle may progress to symmetric ascending paralysis from the legs (hours or days) leading to upper limbs and face with/without numbness or tingling
■ Loss of deep tendon reflexes (areflexia)
■ Difficulty with eye movements; double vision
■ Difficulty with swallowing; drooling
■ Loss of pain and temperature sensation
■ Loss of proprioception (position sense)
■ Sinus tachycardia or bradycardia and cardiac dysrhythmias
■ Orthostatic hypotension; HTN
■ Absence of fever
■ Excessive diaphoresis
■ Seizures
■ Bowel and bladder retention or incontinence

- Changes in vital capacity and negative inspiratory force → respiratory arrest
- ↑ pulmonary secretions
- ↑ protein in CSF (100–1000 mg/dL)
- SIADH
- Residual damage possibly occurring after the acute phase

Diagnostic Tests

- Lumbar puncture and CF analysis
- EMG and nerve conduction velocity studies
- CBC, PFTs, and ABGs

Management

- Assess respiratory status and ABGs.
- Provide early respiratory support, including mechanical ventilation or tracheostomy.
- Assess neurological function—start with lower extremities.
- ECG and BP monitoring.
- Administer antihypertensive or vasopressors to maintain BP within normal limits.
- Insert indwelling Foley catheter if incontinent.
- Provide enteral feedings and nutritional support.
- Active and passive range of motion, physical or occupational therapy.
- Corticosteroids may be tried but generally not effective.
- Provide DVT prophylaxis.
- Administer IVIGs at 400 mg/kg for 5 days.
- Plasmapheresis—40-50 mL/kg plasma exchange four times over a week.
- Provide DVT and peptic ulcer prophylaxis.
- Provide short- and long-term rehabilitation, physical therapy, and occupational therapy consultations.

NEURO

Bacterial Meningitis

Bacterial meningitis is an inflammation that involves the arachnoid and pia mater of the brain, the subarachnoid space, and the CSF.

Pathophysiology

- Bacteria enter the CNS through the bloodstream and crosses the blood-brain barrier or directly enters the bloodstream via penetrating trauma, invasive procedures, cancer, certain drugs, or ruptured cerebral abscess. An upper respiratory infection → bacteria in nasopharynx → bloodstream → CSF subarachnoid space and pia-arachnoid membrane → meninges.
- Purulent exudate → clings to meningeal layers → clogs CSF → vascular congestion and obstruction → cranial nerve dysfunction, hyperemia of meningeal blood vessels, brain tissue edema, ↑ CSF, ↑ WBC in subarachnoid space → acute hydrocephalus and seizures.
- Abnormal stimulation of hypothalamic area → inappropriate ADH production → water retention.

Clinical Presentation

- Symptoms of upper respiratory infection possibly preceding meningeal irritation → severe and unrelenting headache, nausea, vomiting, fever and chills, nuchal rigidity (stiff neck), irritability, malaise, restlessness, myalgia, and tachycardia
- Photophobia and signs of ↑ ICP
- Problems with memory; ↓ LOC; disorientation to person, place, and year; abnormal eye movements → coma, delirium, and seizures
- Kernig's sign: Inability to extend the leg at the knee when the thigh is flexed
- Brudzinski's sign: Flexion of the hip and knee when the patient's neck is flexed

Complications

- Septic emboli and septic shock with vascular dysfunction, or disseminated intravascular coagulation
- Fluid and electrolyte imbalances

- Seizures and hemiparesis
- Cranial nerve (CN) dysfunction: CN III, IV, VI, VII, VIII
- Hydrocephalus and cerebral edema
- ↑ ICP → herniation of the brain

Diagnostic Tests

- Lumbar puncture, culture, and assessment of CSF and pressure → ↑ CSF pressure and protein, ↓ glucose (CSF pressure >180 mm Hg is indicative of bacterial meningitis)
- CBC, especially ↑ WBC
- Blood cultures
- Serum electrolytes, especially Na (dilutional hyponatremia)
- CT scan or MRI if ↑ ICP, or brain abscess or hydrocephalus

Management

- Maintain respiratory isolation until pathogen not cultured in nasopharynx (usually 24 hours after antibiotic treatment).
- Monitor neurological status, cranial nerve function, and vital signs every 1–2 hours. Check pupils, LOC, and motor activity.
- Assess vascular function for signs of septic emboli.
- Ensure ↓ environmental stimuli, quiet environment, and ↓ exposure to lights.
- Administer corticosteroids to decrease inflammation.
- Administer anticonvulsants for seizures.
- Administer antipyretics for fever.
- Administer analgesia for headache.
- Administer hyperosmolar agents for cerebral edema.
- Insert surgical shunt if hydrocephalus is present.
- Consider the following antibiotic therapy:
  - Cefotaxime (Claforan)
  - Ceftazidime (Ceptaz, Fortaz)
  - Ceftriaxone (Rocephin)
  - Vancomycin
  - Meropenem (Merrem)

Assess CSF analysis, gram stain, and cultures for antibiotic sensitivity.

NEURO

Seizure Disorder

A seizure disorder is a temporary, abnormal, sudden, excessive, uncontrolled electrical discharge of neurons of the cerebral cortex. Status epilepticus (SE), which denotes continuous seizure activity, is a medical emergency.

Pathophysiology

Repetitive depolarization of hyperactive hypersensitive brain cells → abnormal electrical activity in the brain.

Risk factors for seizure disorder include

- Epilepsy
- Drug or alcohol abuse
- Drug toxicity (aminophylline)
- Recent head injury
- Infection
- Headache
- Acute metabolic disturbances (hypoglycemia, hyponatremia, hypocalcemia, renal failure)
- CVA
- CNS infection (meningitis, encephalitis)
- CNS trauma or tumor
- Hypoxemia
- Fever (children)
- HTN
- Allergic reaction
- Eclampsia related to pregnancy

Clinical Presentation

- From simple staring to prolonged convulsions
- Brief loss of memory, sparkling or flashes, and sensing of an unpleasant odor
- Classified as motor, sensory, autonomic, emotional, or cognitive
- Aura occurring prior to the seizure along with tachycardia
- Alternation in mental state; confusion or dazed state
- Tonic or clonic movements

- Loss of consciousness
- Déjà vu or jamais vu (any familiar situation that is not recognized by the observer)

The clinical presentation of seizure disorder depends on the type of seizure.

Complications

- Pulmonary edema
- Pulmonary aspiration
- Cardiac dysrhythmias
- HTN or hypotension
- Hyperthermia
- Hyperglycemia/hypoglycemia
- Hypoxia
- Dehydration
- Myoglobinuria
- Oral or musculoskeletal injuries

Diagnostic Tests

- Electroencephalogram (EEG)
- CT scan, MRI, or PET to rule out cerebral lesions
- Serum drug screen to rule out drug or alcohol intoxication
- Serum electrolytes, BUN, calcium, magnesium, glucose
- CBC
- ECG to detect cardiac arrhythmias
- ABGs or pulse oximetry

Management

- Administer fast-acting anticonvulsants:
  - Lorazepam (Ativan) 0.1 mg/kg at <2 mg/min IV
  - Diazepam (Valium) 5–10 mg IV
- Administer long-acting anticonvulsants:
  - Phenytoin (Dilantin): 20 mg/kg at <50 mg/min IV
  - Phenobarbital (Luminal): 100–320 mg IV
  - Fosphenytoin (Cerebyx): 20 mg/kg at 150 mg/min

NEURO

- Propofol (Diprivan): dosage per anesthesiologist
  - Midazolam (Versed): dosage per anesthesiologist
- Identify precipitating factors and preceding aura.
- Ensure patient safety (pad side rails, bed at lowest position).
- Prevent Wernicke-Korsakoff syndrome; administer thiamine 100 mg IV and 50 mL of 50% glucose if chronic alcohol ingestion or hypoglycemia is present.
- Keep oral or nasal airway or endotracheal tube (ETT) at bedside.
- During seizure:
  - Observe seizure type, point of origin, and spread of seizure activity
  - Note length of time of seizure
  - Note automatisms, such as lip smacking and repeated swallowing
  - Assess LOC, bowel and bladder incontinence, and tongue biting
  - Avoid restraining patient
  - Avoid forcing airway into patient's mouth when jaws clenched
  - Avoid use of tongue blade
  - Maintain patent airway during seizure
- During postictal state (after seizure):
  - Assess vital signs closely; provide ECG monitoring
  - Monitor oxygenation and respiratory status (ABGs, SpO_2, breath sounds)
  - Turn patient to side-lying position; administer O_2 therapy; suction prn
  - Check level of orientation and ability to speak (patient usually sleeps afterward)
  - Note headache and signs of increased intracranial pressure
  - Check pupil size, eye deviations, and response to auditory and tactile stimuli
  - Note paralysis or weakness of arms or legs

Acute Gastrointestinal Bleeding

Causes of upper GI (UGI) bleeding include:

- Gastric or duodenal ulcers including stress ulcers; may be nonsteroidal anti-inflammatory drug (NSAIDs) related
- Peptic ulcer disease, gastritis, or esophagitis
- Esophagogastric varices
- Mallory-Weiss tear
- Neoplasms
- Liver disorders

Causes of lower GI bleeding include:

- Diverticulosis
- Infectious colitis
- Bowel disease or trauma
- Neoplasm
- Hemorrhoids or anorectal disorders

Pathophysiology

- Constriction of peripheral arteries → ↓ blood flow to skin and kidneys → renal failure; ↓ blood flow to GI tract → mesenteric insufficiency → bowel infarction and liver necrosis; ↓ blood flow to coronary arteries → myocardial infarction (MI), pulmonary edema, heart failure, and dysrhythmias; ↓ blood flow to brain → confusion, anxiety, restlessness, stupor, and coma.
- Acute massive GI bleed → ↓ blood volume → ↓ cardiac output → ↓ BP, ↑ HR → hypovolemic shock and multiple organ dysfunction.
- Metabolic acidosis and lactic acid accumulation → anoxia and respiratory failure.

Clinical Presentation

- Hematemesis: Bright red or brown, coffee-ground emesis
- Melena: Black, tarry stools
- Hematochezia: Maroon-colored stools or bright red blood
- Hypotension: May be orthostatic, light headedness, fainting

GI

- Tachycardia: ↓ pulse pressure, capillary refill sluggish
- Cardiac dysrhythmias
- Tachypnea, shortness of breath, chest pain
- Pallor, apprehension, confusion, lethargy, weakness
- ↓ urine output, ↑ urine concentration
- ↑ bowel sounds, diarrhea
- Stupor and coma if large blood loss
- Multiple organ dysfunction if severe blood loss and hypovolemic shock

Diagnostic Tests

- CBC, platelets, and coagulation studies
- Serum chemistries, liver function tests, and blood urea nitrogen/creatinine ratio (if >36 → GI bleed if no renal insufficiency)
- Arterial blood gases (ABGs) or pulse oximetry
- UGI series
- Abdominal x-ray or CT of abdomen
- Barium enema
- GI bleeding scan
- Endoscopy
- Colonoscopy or sigmoidoscopy

Management

- Monitor vital signs and hemodynamics (central venous pressure [CVP], pulmonary artery pressure [PAP]). Note ↓ BP, ↑ HR, ↓ CVP and cardiac output.
- Monitor for cardiac dysrhythmias.
- Assess respiratory status and ABGs or pulse oximetry. Administer O_2 via cannula, mask, or mechanical ventilation. Assess for signs of hypoxia.
- Insert nasogastric (NG) tube and set at low intermittent suction. Lavage as necessary. Assess color and amount of drainage. Note bright red to coffee-ground drainage. Keep patient NPO if active bleeding. Start clear liquids when bleeding stops.
- Assess bowel sounds; assess abdomen for distention and palpate for pain.
- Administer IV fluids, colloids, crystalloids, blood, and blood products.

- Note amount and color of feces. Hematest stool prn.
- Insert Foley catheter. Monitor intake and output. Assess fluid and electrolyte balance.
- Administer histamine blockers or proton pump inhibitors. Consider misoprostol (prostaglandin analog), anticholinergics, or mucosal protective agents.
- Administer IV or intra-arterial vasopressin with caution.
- If coagulopathy is present ($\uparrow$ partial thromboplastin time [PTT]), administer vitamin K and fresh frozen plasma.
- Administer tranexamic acid (Cyklokapron) if excessive bleeding and decreased fibrinolysis.
- A specific protocol of medications is ordered if patient is *Helicobacter pylori* positive.
- Provide emotional support to patient and family. Relieve anxiety and pain.
- Prepare patient for possible endoscopic or surgical procedures:
  - Laser phototherapy
  - Endoscopic thermal or injection therapy
  - Intra-arterial embolization
  - Vagotomy, pyloroplasty, or total or partial gastrectomy

Complications

- Gastric perforation $\rightarrow$ sudden and severe generalized abdominal pain with rebound tenderness and board-like abdominal rigidity
- Reduced cardiac output, including hypovolemic shock
- Nausea, vomiting, and diarrhea
- Altered nutritional status with nutritional deficits; aspiration
- Infection; fever, $\uparrow$ WBC and $\uparrow$ HR

Esophageal Varices

Esophageal varices are dilated, distended, tortuous veins in the esophagus. They may also occur in the proximal stomach. These varices are most commonly due to portal hypertension (>10 mm Hg) secondary to hepatic cirrhosis caused by the consumption of large amounts of alcohol.

Pathophysiology

Impaired liver structure and function → ↑ resistance to portal blood flow at portal vena and inferior vena cava and ↑ pressure in the liver → ↑ portal venous pressure (portal hypertension) → collateral circulation from the liver to the veins of the esophagus, spleen, intestines, and stomach → engorged and dilated blood vessels → esophagogastric varices → rupture → massive hemorrhage → death.

Clinical Presentation

- Vomiting of blood (hematemesis) or massive bleeding (hematochezia)
- Tachycardia; ↓ BP; cool, clammy skin; decreased urine output
- Bright red to black stools, indicating blood in feces
- Abdominal pain and weakness
- Other signs of upper GI bleeding

Diagnostic Tests

- CBC, serum chemistries, and liver enzymes
- Platelet count, prothrombin time (PT)/PTT, and fibrinogen
- Type and crossmatch for possible blood administration
- Endoscopy
- Liver biopsy
- Splenoportography, hepatoportography, or celiac angiography

Management

- Administer antibiotics to prevent/control infection.
- Provide nutritional supplementation.
- Administer octreotide (Sandostatin) infusion to ↓ portal pressure.
- Initiate arterial or central line infusion of vasopressin (Pitressin). Use with caution; → myocardial or mesenteric ischemia and infarction due to vasoconstriction.
- Insert esophagogastric balloon tamponade.
- Prepare patient for endoscopic injection therapy (sclerotherapy).
- Prepare patient endoscopic variceal ligation/banding or apply hemoclips.

- Initiate treatment with heater probe, laser therapy, or electrocoagulation.
- Prepare patient transjugular intrahepatic portosystemic shunt (TIPS).
- Prepare patient portacaval shunt, mesocaval shunt, or splenorenal shunt.
- Refer to assessment and management of patients with GI bleeding.

Esophagogastric Balloon Tamponade

- Esophagogastric balloon tamponade is used to control esophageal variceal bleeding through use of the Sengstaken-Blakemore tube or Minnesota tube. A Linton-Nachlas tube is used for isolated gastric hemorrhage, such as with gastric varices. The balloons apply direct pressure to the varices → ↓ blood flow.
- The Sengstaken-Blakemore tube has 3 lumens: gastric aspiration, esophageal balloon inflation, and gastric balloon inflation. The Minnesota tube has a 4th lumen for esophageal aspiration. The inflation of the balloons is as follows:
    - The esophageal balloon is inflated to 25–35 mm Hg pressure for a maximum of 36 hours.
    - The gastric balloon is inflated to 500 mL of air or as specified by manufacturer for a maximum of 72 hours.
    - 1 to 3 lbs of pressure is used for tension on the balloons.
    - One port is connected to intermittent suction.

Postsurgical Management

- Confirm placement by chest x-ray.
- Assess airway patency.
- Scissors should be placed at the bedside for cutting the balloons if airway obstructed.
- Position patient in high-Fowler's position or on left side.
- Provide frequent oral and nares care and oral suction.
- Monitor gastric and esophageal output. The balloons may be deflated every 8 to 12 hours to decompress the esophagus and stomach. Assess for bleeding.
- The esophageal balloon must be deflated before the gastric balloon to prevent upward migration of the esophageal balloon → airway occlusion.
- To discontinue tamponade therapy, gradually decrease esophageal balloon pressure. Observe for bleeding. If no further bleeding, then deflate the gastric balloon. If no further bleeding within the following 4 hours, the tube may be removed. Continue to monitor for bleeding.

Complications

- Esophageal erosion and rupture
- Pulmonary aspiration
- Balloon migration
- Nasal necrosis

Institution Specific Care:

_____
_____
_____
_____
_____

Hepatic Failure

Hepatic failure occurs when there is a loss of 60% of hepatocytes. It may be chronic or acute and can lead to hepatic encephalopathy. Causes of hepatic failure include:

- Cirrhosis of the liver
- Hepatitis A, hepatitis B, hepatitis C, and Epstein-Barr virus
- IV drug use, cocaine use, and acetaminophen toxicity
- Repeated environmental and hepatotoxin exposure
- Malignancy
- Hypoperfusion of the liver
- Metabolic disorders: Reye's syndrome, Wilson's disease
- Malnutrition, diabetes mellitus, chronic cholestatic disease, and hypertriglyceridemia
- Postoperatively: jejunoileal bypass, partial hepatectomy, liver transplant failure

Pathophysiology

- Severe liver impairment such as necrosis or ↓ blood supply to liver → toxic substances accumulating in the blood.
- Impaired bilirubin conjugation, ↓ clotting factors, ↓ glucose synthesis, ↓ lactate clearance → jaundice, coagulopathies, hypoglycemia, and metabolic acidosis.
- Decreased macrophages in liver → ↑ risk of infection and spleen enlargement.

- Hypoalbuminemia, fluid and electrolyte imbalances, acute portal hypertension → development of ascites.
- Ineffective fat metabolism → ↓ bile salt production.
- Cirrhosis: Fibrotic tissue replaces healthy liver tissue.
- Fatty liver disease: Fatty cells replace healthy liver tissue.
- Hepatic failure may progress to hepatic encephalopathy.

Clinical Presentation

- Jaundice, ascites, edema, and pruritus
- Malnutrition, nausea, vomiting, and anorexia
- Weakness, fatigue, and confusion
- Hyperventilation, respiratory alkalosis, dyspnea, pleural effusion, and hypoxemia
- Hypokalemia and hypo- or hypernatremia
- Palmar erythema, spider nevi, and bruising
- Asterixis: Liver flap (patient extends arms → wrist dorsiflexes downward involuntarily)
- Metabolic acidosis, hypoglycemia, hypokalemia, and hyponatremia
- Gallstones, malnutrition, light-colored stools, and dark urine
- Diarrhea and steatorrhea (fatty, greasy, foul-smelling stools)
- Hepatic encephalopathy: Drowsiness, confusion, delirium or coma, inappropriate behavior, fetor hepaticus (breath odor), and day-night reversal

Diagnostic Tests

- CT scan or ultrasound
- Serum chemistries, bilirubin, and albumin
- AST, APT, ALT, and cholesterol
- Ammonia levels
- CBC and platelets
- ABGs or pulse oximetry
- PT, PTT, plasmin, plasminogen, fibrin, and fibrin-split products
- Urinalysis, urine bilirubin, and urine urobilinogen

Management

- Administer lactulose orally or rectally. Administer Neomycin orally or rectally if not contraindicated.
- Administer diuretics such as furosemide (Lasix) if ascites present. Monitor intake and output. Prepare patient for paracentesis.
- Measure abdominal girth; weigh daily.
- Monitor for cardiac dysrhythmias.
- Provide stress ulcer prophylaxis. Elevate head of bed 20°–30°. Assess for signs of GI bleeding.
- Administer vitamin K and platelets. Avoid frequent venipunctures.
- Treat fever and control BP.
- Correct fluid and electrolyte imbalances. Prevent and correct hypokalemia, which increases renal ammonia production → ammonia across the blood-brain barrier.
- Prevent infection. Administer prophylactic antibiotics. Consider rifaximin (Xifaxan).
- Assess neurological status, level of consciousness, Glasgow Coma Scale score, and response to verbal and noxious stimuli.
- Assess for signs of increased intracranial pressure (ICP). Administer mannitol.
- Assess respiratory status, and monitor ABGs or pulse oximetry. Correct hypercapnia and hypoxemia via O_2 administration or mechanical ventilation.
- Provide continuous renal replacement therapy (CRRT) if renal failure present.
- Avoid benzodiazepines and other sedatives that may mask symptoms. Consider oxazepam (Serax), diazepam (Valium), or lorazepam (Ativan) if sedation is required.
- Use physical restraints as necessary. Provide reality orientation. Institute measures for patient safety.
- Administer medications with caution. Adjust dosage per liver function tests.
- Provide a low-protein, low-sodium diet. Restrict fluids as necessary. Consider enteral feeding or total parenteral nutrition (TPN) if oral intake insufficient. Assess for hypoglycemia. Monitor serum albumin, electrolytes, and liver function tests.

- Prevent intravascular volume depletion through IV fluids, colloids, and crystalloids. Avoid lactated Ringer's solution.
- Avoid hazards of immobility. Provide meticulous skin care.
- Monitor ammonia levels (80–110 µg/dl or 47–65 µmol/L [SI units]).
- Provide comfort measures and emotional support.
- Prepare patient for TIPS to ↓ portal hypertension, prevent rebleeding from varices, and ↓ formation of ascites.
- Prepare patient for liver transplantation if necessary.

Complications

- Cerebral edema and increased ICP, and low cerebral perfusion pressure
- Cardiac dysrhythmias and coagulopathy
- Respiratory depression, acute respiratory failure, and respiratory arrest
- Sepsis and circulatory failure
- Acute renal failure
- Hypoxemia, metabolic acidosis, and electrolyte imbalances
- Hypoglycemia
- GI bleeding
- Hepatic failure may progress to hepatic encephalopathy → death. Hepatic encephalopathy is divided into the following types:
  - Type A: hepatic encephalopathy associated with acute liver failure
  - Type B: hepatic encephalopathy caused by portal-systemic shunting without associated intrinsic liver disease
  - Type C: hepatic encephalopathy associated with cirrhosis
- The severity of hepatic encephalopathy is evaluated according to the following grades:
  - Grade 1: Euphoria or anxiety, shortened attention span
  - Grade 2: Lethargy, apathy, subtle personality change, inappropriate behavior, minimal disorientation to time or place
  - Grade 3: Somnolence to semistupor, responds to verbal stimuli, confusion
  - Grade 4: Coma, unresponsive to stimuli

Pancreatitis

Pancreatitis is an inflammation of the pancreas that can be categorized into edematous interstitial pancreatitis and acute necrotizing pancreatitis. 10%–20% of cases of pancreatitis are idiopathic and have no etiologic factor. Causes of pancreatitis include:

- Alcoholism
- Gallstones, biliary disease, and hypertriglyceridemia
- Infection (e.g., mumps, ischemia)
- Blunt abdominal trauma and surgical trauma
- Hyperparathyroidism, hypercalcemia, and hyperthyroidism
- Systemic lupus erythematosus and vasculitis
- Medications such as glucocoticoids, sulfanomides, tetracyclines, NSAIDs, furosemide, hydrochlorothiazide, and estrogen

Pathophysiology

- Trypsinogen is converted to trypsin (pancreatic enzymes) → destruction of ductal tissue and pancreatic cells → autodigestion and fibrosis of the pancreas.
- An increase in capillary permeability → leakage of fluid into the interstitium → edema, hypovolemia, hemorrhage, pancreatic, and adipose tissue necrosis → third spacing of fluids → systemic inflammatory response syndrome (SIRS).
- Obstruction of the pancreatic duct → reflux of bile into the pancreas → enzyme reaction.
- Drugs and toxins → autodigestion and inflammation.

Clinical Presentation

- Severe knife-like midepigastric or midabdominal pain that may radiate to the back; onset of pain is frequently 24–48 hours after a heavy meal or alcohol ingestion; pain may also be diffuse and difficult to localize
- Nausea and vomiting
- Fever, diaphoresis, and weakness
- Tachypnea, ↓ BP, ↑ HR, and other symptoms of hypovolemic shock
- Hypoactive or absent bowel sounds, and abdominal tenderness and distention

- Ascites and jaundice if illness severe
- Pancreatic hemorrhage → Grey Turner's sign (gray-blue discoloration of the flank) or Cullen's sign (discoloration of the umbilical region)
- Palpable abdominal mass if pseudocyst or abscess present
- Hypocalcemia and hyperlipidemia

Diagnostic Tests

- Serum amylase (30–220 U/L [SI units] normal) and/or lipase (0–160 U/L [SI units] normal) ≥3 times the upper limit of normal
- Abdominal flat plate or ultrasound of abdomen, CT, MRI, and endoscopic cholangiopancreatography
- Chest x-ray to detect pleural effusions
- Serum chemistries, including ↓ calcium, ↓ magnesium, ↑ bilirubin, ↑ glucose, ↓ potassium, ↑ liver enzymes, ↓ albumin, and ↑ triglycerides
- Urinalysis and ↑ urinary amylase (6.5–48.1 U/hr [SI units])
- CBC (↑ WBC, hematocrit and hemoglobin may be ↑ or ↓), PT/PTT, ↑ C-reactive protein
- ABGs to assess for hypoxemia and metabolic acidosis

Management

- Administer analgesics; position patient in knee-chest position.
- Consider prophylactic antibiotics. For necrotizing pancreatitis, administer imipenem-cilastatin (Primaxin) for its high concentration of the drug in the pancreas.
- Assess fluid and electrolyte balance. Note hypokalemia or hypocalcemia. Administer IV fluids, crystalloids, and colloids. Monitor intake and output.
- Assess nutritional status. Keep patient NPO initially. Consider TPN, or gastric or jejunal enteral feedings. Stress ulcer prophylaxis.
- Insert NG tube if vomiting, obstruction, or gastric distention is present. Provide frequent oral care.
- Assess for metabolic acidosis.
- Assess respiratory status and monitor ABGs or venous oxygen saturation. Administer O_2 as needed.
- Administer insulin if elevated blood glucose levels exist.

- Assess abdomen for distention, rigidity, ascites, and increasing pain or rebound tenderness; auscultate bowel sounds and measure abdominal girth.
- Treat fever and monitor WBC count.
- Assess vital signs. Monitor for cardiac arrhythmias.
- Prepare patient for surgical debridement or pancreatic resection for necrotizing pancreatitis or drainage of pancreatic pseudocyst or abscess.

Complications

- Pancreatic abscess or pseudocyst formation, and bowel infarction
- Acute lung injury (ALI), pleural effusion, atelectasis, pneumonia, pneumonitis, hypoxemia, respiratory failure, and acute respiratory distress syndrome
- Hypotension, pericardial effusion, myocardial depression, cardiac dysrhythmias, and disseminated intravascular coagulation
- Acute renal failure, acute tubular necrosis, and azotemia
- Hepatic dysfunction, obstructive jaundice, and paralytic ileus
- Stress ulcers and esophageal varices → GI hemorrhage
- Systemic inflammatory response syndrome
- Severe hemorrhage and shock
- Multiorgan failure, sepsis, and death

Peritonitis

Peritonitis is the inflammation of the peritoneum, the serous membrane lining the abdominal cavity and covering the viscera. It may be localized or generalized. Peritonitis is an example of acute abdomen.

Pathophysiology

Inflammation, bacterial infection, ischemia, tumor, and trauma → leakage of contents from the abdominal organs into the abdominal cavity → tissue edema → fluid in peritoneal cavity.

Clinical Presentation

- Abdominal pain that increases with movement such as coughing and flexing the hips; rebound tenderness, guarding, and abdominal rigidity (washboard abdomen); Blumberg's sign: Pressing a hand on the abdomen elicits pain, but pain increases when releasing the hand as the peritoneum moves back into place
- Air and fluid in the bowel
- Abdominal distention, hyperactive → hypoactive bowel sounds → paralytic ileus
- Nausea and vomiting
- Fever and ↑ HR
- Cloudy effluent if on peritoneal dialysis

Diagnostic Tests

- CBC: assess for leukocytosis, and ↓ hemoglobin and hematocrit
- Serum chemistries
- Abdominal x-ray
- Peritoneal lavage or peritoneal aspiration, and culture and sensitivity studies of peritoneal fluid or peritoneal effluent

Complications

- Fluid and electrolyte imbalance, ↓ CVP, hypovolemia → shock → acute renal failure
- Intestinal obstruction due to bowel adhesions
- Peritoneal abscess
- Sepsis

Management

- Administer antibiotics. Obtain blood cultures to assess for sepsis.
- Obtain peritoneal effluent cultures.
- Provide fluid and electrolyte replacement. Monitor intake and output.
- Administer analgesics and antiemetics. Place patient on side with knees flexed.

- Monitor vital signs. Assess for ↓ BP and ↑ HR. Provide cardiac monitoring.
- Assess respiratory status. Administer O_2 as indicated by ABGs or pulse oximetry.
- Assess abdomen for pain and distention. Auscultate bowel sounds.
- Perform surgery to remove infected material and correct the cause.

Crohn's Disease

Crohn's disease is an inflammatory bowel disease that may occur anywhere along the GI tract. The terminal ileum and proximal large intestine are usually involved.

Pathophysiology

Chronic inflammation → edema and thickening of intestinal mucosa → ulcers forming in the intestines → fistulas, fissures, and abscesses → thickening of bowel wall → narrowing of intestinal lumen → scar tissue and granulomas → weepy edematous intestines.

Clinical Presentation

- Lower right quadrant abdominal pain that usually occurs after meals
- Abdominal tenderness and spasm
- Chronic diarrhea and steatorrhea (excessive fat in stool)
- Weight loss, anorexia, malnutrition, and anemia

Diagnostic Tests

- Sigmoidoscopy, colonoscopy, intestinal biopsies, and testing for *Clostridium difficile*
- Stool analysis for occult blood and steatorrhea, and stool culture and sensitivity (C&S)
- UGI series or endoscopy, and barium enema
- Abdominal x-rays and CT, MRI, or ultrasound of the abdomen
- CBC, erythrocyte sedimentation rate (ESR), and C-reactive protein
- Serum chemistries, including albumin, protein, and calcium, and liver function tests

Management

- Administer aminosalicylates:
  - Sulfasalazine (Azulfidine)
  - Mesalamine or mesalazine (5-ASA, Asacol, Pentasa)
  - Balsalazide (Colazal)
  - Olsalazine (Dipentum)
- Administer corticosteroids:
  - Prednisone or hydrocortisone
  - Prednisolone or methylprednisolone
  - Beclomethasone or budesonide
- Consider administration of antibiotics.
- Administer analgesics for pain.
- Assess vital signs for ↑ HR and fever, and assess for pallor.
- Assess bowel sounds, and examine abdomen for distention and tenderness.
- Assess number and frequency of stools, and test stool for occult blood and parasites.
- Administer IV fluids to correct fluid and electrolyte imbalance.
- Maintain NPO with TPN, or provide diet high in protein and calories with vitamins and iron.
- Administer bulk hydrophilic agents.
- Prepare patient for surgery as needed (partial or complete colectomy with ileostomy of anastomosis).

Ulcerative Colitis

Ulcerative colitis is an inflammatory autoimmune disease of the bowel. It is characterized by ulcers or open sores in the colon that affect the mucosal layer. The patient experiences remissions and exacerbations with an increased risk of colorectal cancer.

Pathophysiology

Multiple ulcerations of the colon → bleeding → mucosa becomes edematous and inflamed → abscesses → narrowing, shortening and thickening of the bowel.

Clinical Presentation

- Diarrhea mixed with blood and mucus (as many as 10–20 liquid stools/day) and an urgent need to defecate
- Crampy abdominal pain in the left lower quadrant and rebound tenderness in the right lower quadrant
- Intermittent tenesmus: Constant feeling of the need to defecate with little or no fecal output
- Rectal bleeding
- Pallor, anemia, and fatigue
- Anorexia, weight loss, vomiting, and dehydration
- Fever and tachycardia

Diagnostic Tests

- Sigmoidoscopy, colonoscopy, intestinal biopsies, and testing for *Clostridium difficile*
- Stool analysis for occult blood and steatorrhea, and stool C&S
- UGI series or endoscopy, and barium enema
- Abdominal x-rays and CT, MRI, or ultrasound of the abdomen
- CBC, ESR, and C-reactive protein
- Serum chemistries, including albumin, protein, and calcium, and liver function tests

Management

- Assess vital signs for ↑ HR, ↓ BP, ↑ RR, and fever, and assess for pallor.
- Assess skin in the perianal area for redness and skin breakdown.
- Assess bowel sounds, and examine abdomen for distention and tenderness.
- Assess number and frequency of stools, and test stool for occult blood and parasites.
- Administer IV fluids to correct fluid and electrolyte imbalance.
- Maintain NPO with TPN, or provide diet high in protein and calories with vitamins and iron.
- Administer bulk hydrophilic agents.
- Administer antibiotics, such as metronidazole (Flagyl).

- Administer aminosalicylates:
  - Sulfasalazine (Azulfidine)
  - Mesalamine or mesalazine (5-ASA, Asacol, Pentasa)
  - Balsalazide (Colazal)
  - Olsalazine (Dipentum)
- Administer corticosteroids:
  - Prednisone or hydrocortisone
  - Prednisolone or methylprednisolone
  - Beclomethasone or budesonide
- Administer GI anti-inflammatories/monoclonal antibodies:
  - Infliximab (Remicade)
  - Visilizumab (Nuvion)
- Administer immunosuppressants:
  - Mercaptopurine (6-MP)
  - Azathioprine (Imuran, Azasan)
  - Methotrexate (Amethopterin)
  - Tacrolimus (Prograf)
- Administer analgesics, sedatives, and antidiarrheals as needed.
- Prepare patient for surgery as needed (total colectomy with ileostomy, continent ileostomy, or bowel resection).

Complications

- Toxic megacolon → colonic distention → fever, abdominal pain and distention, vomiting, and fatigue (does not respond to medical management within 24–72 hours)
- Intestinal perforation and bleeding
- Pyelonephritis and nephrolithiasis
- Malignant neoplasms

Small Bowel Obstruction

SBO is a mechanical or functional obstruction of the small intestines. The normal transit of the products of digestion through the intestines is blocked.

Causes

- Adhesions and hernias
- Crohn's disease
- Benign or malignant tumors
- Foreign bodies

Pathophysiology

- Intestinal contents, gas, and fluid accumulate above the obstruction → abdominal distention and fluid retention → ↓ venous and arteriolar capillary pressure → edema, congestion, and necrosis of the intestine → rupture or perforation of the intestinal wall → peritonitis.
- SBO may also lead to intestinal strangulation.
- Reflex vomiting also occurs → ↓ H$^+$ and K$^+$ → metabolic acidosis, and ↓ H$_2$O and ↓ Na$^+$ → dehydration → hypovolemic shock.
- Obstruction may resolve spontaneously.

Clinical Presentation

- Crampy, colicky, wave-like central or midabdominal pain
- No bowel movement and absence of flatus → abdominal distention → bowel ischemia or perforation
- Nausea and vomiting → dehydration (drowsiness, malaise, and parched tongue and mucous membranes) and electrolyte imbalances → hypovolemic shock
- Possible aspiration of vomitus (vomitus may be fecal in nature)

Diagnostic Tests

- Abdominal x-ray; CT scan and ultrasound of the abdomen
- Contrast enema or small bowel series
- Colonoscopy and laparoscopy
- CBC and serum chemistries

Management

- Insert NG tube and connect to low intermittent suction; assess color and amount of drainage.

- Administer IV fluids, and assess fluid and electrolyte balance.
- Monitor nutritional status. Monitor intake and output.
- Assess abdomen for bowel sounds, pain, and distention.
- Administer analgesics for pain.
- Prepare patient for surgery as indicated to relieve the obstruction.

Morbid Obesity

Morbid obesity is defined as a body mass index (BMI) >30–40 kg/m^2, a body weight twice the person's ideal body weight, or a body weight more than 100 lbs. greater than the ideal body weight.

Persons who are morbidly obese are at a higher risk for:

- Diabetes mellitus
- Cardiovascular disease, including stroke and hypertension
- Hypertrophic cardiomyopathy
- Hyperlipidemia
- Gallbladder disease
- Osteoarthritis
- Obstructive sleep apnea
- Obesity hypoventilation syndrome
- Certain cancers (uterine, breast, colorectal, kidney, and gallbladder)

Psychosocial problems may also co-exist:

- Low self-esteem
- Impaired body image
- Depression
- Social anxiety/isolation

Management

Pharmacological Management
- Sibutramine HCL (Meridia).
- Orlistat (Xenical).

Surgical Management
- Bariatric surgical techniques include those based on gastric restriction and those combining gastric restriction and malabsorption. They

GI

include gastric bypass (Roux-en-Y), gastric banding, vertical-banded gastroplasty, and biliopancreatic diversion (BPD).

- Gastric restriction surgeries use staples or banding to reduce the stomach size to 15 mL.
- Vertical-banded gastroplasty (Mason procedure or stomach stapling) creates a pouch, and a band is placed at the lower end of the pouch → creation of a stoma → emptying into the small intestine.
- Circumgastric (adjustable) banding limits the stomach size through the placement of an inflatable band around the fundus of the stomach. This may be done laparoscopically.
- BPD (Scopinaro procedure) has been replaced by duodenal switch (BPD/DS). In BPD/DS, part of the stomach is resected and the distal part of the small intestine is connected to the stomach pouch, bypassing the duodenum and jejunum.
- Gastric bypass surgery (most commonly performed operation for weight loss) creates a stomach pouch that is connected to the distal small intestine.

Postoperative Management

Standard postoperative care should be provided, with the following special attention:

- Administer analgesics for pain.
- Vigilantly assess respiratory status. Patient may need long-term ventilatory support with use of tracheostomy.
- Elevate head of bed 30° to reduce weight of adipose tissue on the diaphragm.
- Encourage early ambulation; turn and position frequently with use of trapeze on the bed.
- Assess for skin breakdown especially within skin folds.
- When starting diet, provide 6 small feedings/day (totaling 600–800 calories); encourage fluids to prevent dehydration.
- Provide deep vein thrombosis (DVT) prophylaxis.

Complications may include:

- Bleeding from surgical site or internally
- Thromboembolism and pulmonary embolism
- Atelectasis and pneumonia

- Bowel obstruction, incisional or ventral hernias, wound dehiscence, and slow wound healing
- Infection: Respiratory, urinary, wound, or sepsis
- Anastomosis leak → peritonitis
- Abdominal compartment syndrome
- Nausea, vomiting, gastric dumping syndrome (↑ HR, nausea, tremor, dizziness, fatigue, abdominal cramps, and diarrhea), and diarrhea or constipation
- Fluid and electrolyte imbalances
- Gallstones, nutritional deficiencies, electrolyte imbalance, anemia, and weight gain (long-term complications)

Gastrointestinal Surgery

Esophagectomy is the removal of the entire esophagus and part of the stomach and lymph nodes in the surrounding area.

Whipple procedure or pancreaticoduodenectomy is the removal of the head of the pancreas, duodenum, part of the jejunum, common bile duct, gallbladder, and part of the stomach.

Complications

- Atelectasis, pneumonia, and respiratory failure
- DVT and pulmonary embolism
- UGI bleeding
- Gastritis, esophagitis, and dumping syndrome
- Anastomotic leak: Tachycardia, tachypnea, fever, abdominal pain, anxiety and restlessness, subcutaneous emphysema (crepitus), and sepsis

Management

- Provide standard postoperative care, including administration of analgesics and provision of pulmonary care.
- Assess for GI bleeding.
- Provide DVT prophylaxis. Encourage early ambulation.

Percutaneous transjugular intrahepatic portosystemic shunt (TIPS) is an interventional procedure to decrease portal hypertension and reduce complications from high hepatic pressures. A catheter is placed in a hepatic vein, and a stent is placed in the liver parenchyma. Postprocedure, observe for bleeding due to hepatic or portal vein puncture, puncture of the biliary tree, bile duct trauma, and stent migration or thrombosis.

Hematologic and Oncologic Disorders

Disseminated Intravascular Coagulation

DIC is a disorder characterized by massive systemic intravascular activation of coagulation caused by a variety of clinical conditions, including sepsis (Gram + and Gram – infections), severe trauma or burns, and solid or hematologic cancers. It can also be caused by some obstetric conditions, such as placental abruption, amniotic fluid embolism, and placenta previa.

Pathophysiology

- Activation of thrombus → fibrinogen fibrin formation and deposition of fibrin in the microvasculature → an ↑ in platelet aggregation or adhesions → formation of fibrin clots to form → diffuse obstruction of the smaller vessels → progressive organ dysfunction (i.e., renal insufficiency, ARDS, hypotension, circulatory failure, skin necrosis).
- Concurrent with these events, platelets, prothrombin, and fibrinogen are used up → a deficiency of these factors compromising coagulation and predisposing to bleeding.
- The excessive clotting at the microvasculature level activates the fibrinolytic system → production of fibrin degradation products (FDPs) (i.e., fibrin split products) → an anticoagulation effect of FDP with fibrinogen and thrombin → interference with the formation of fibrin clot and decreased platelet function → bleeding → hemorrhagic bleeding.

Clinical Presentation

- Bleeding (purpura, petechiae, eccymosis)
- GI bleeding (hematemesis, melena, tarry stools)
- GU/GYN bleeding (hematuria, menorrhagia in women)
- Wound bleeding
- Bleeding and oozing from puncture sites and around invasive catheters and lines
- Hematoma formation
- Pulmonary hemorrhage
- Large foci of skin necrosis (resulting from tissue injury and necrosis associated with compromised circulation)
- Acrocyonosis (cyanosis of hands and feet)

HEMA/ONCO

- Acute multiorgan dysfunction (characterized by hypotension, oliguria, dyspnea, confusion, convulsions, coma, abdominal pain, diarrhea, and other GI symptoms)
- Angina
- Malaise
- Dyspnea
- Fatigue and weakness
- Headache
- Nausea and vomiting
- Palpitations
- Severe pain in abdomen, back, muscles, joints, and bones
- Sudden vision changes
- Vertigo
- Confusion and anxiety/irritability
- Convulsions
- Coma

Diagnostic Tests
- CBC
- Prothrombin time (PT)/partial thromboplastin time (PTT)
- Fibrinogen level
- Fibrin degradation/ split products
- D-dimer
- Thrombin time
- Anti-thrombin III (AT III)

Management
- Be aware of early signs of impaired tissue perfusion in patients at high risk for DIC (subtle mental status change, hypotension [especially orthostatic]), dyspnea, tachypnea, syncope, decreased urine output.
- Start heparin infusion.
- Replace deficient clotting factors.
- Administer vitamin K and folate.
- Administer platelet infusion.
- Administer fresh frozen plasma (FFP) infusion.
- Administer cryoprecipitate infusion.
- Provide blood transfusion.
- Administer O_2 as needed.
- Provide support to patient and family.

Heparin-Induced Thrombocytopenia

Heparin-induced thrombocytopenia is a transient disorder in which thrombocytopenia (>50% ↓ in platelet count) appears approximately 1 week after exposure to heparin. There is a strong association with venous and arterial blood clot formation.

Pathophysiology

After heparin is administered, an immune complex can form between heparin and specific blood factor (platelet factor 4 [PF4]) that is released by platelets → body viewing this "heparin-PF4" as a foreign body → formation of antibodies against the heparin PF4 complex → antibodies binding to the complex → platelet destruction → disruption of platelets → formation of new blood clot → deep vein thrombosis (DVT), pulmonary embolism (PE), myocardial infarction (MI) or cerebrovascular accident (CVA).

Clinical Presentation

- Signs and symptoms of DVT (pain or tenderness, sudden swelling, discoloration of visible leg veins)
- Signs and symptoms of PE (SOB, change in HR, sharp chest pain, dizziness, anxiety, excessive sweating)
- Severe indicators:
  - Skin changes (bruising or blackening around injection site as well as on fingers and toes, and nipples) ↑ gangrene

Diagnostic Tests

- CBC
- PT/PTT
- PF4 assay
- Platelet activation assay (C-SRA; heparin- induced platelet activation assay)

Management

- Discontinue all heparin products.
- Administer IV direct thrombin inhibitor for anticoagulation:
  - Lepirudin (Refludan)
  - Argatroban (Acova)
  - Bivalirudin (Angiomax)
- CBC: monitor platelet count.

- Once platelet count is normal, initiate Coumadin therapy.
- Provide a complete skin and neurovascular assessment.
- Provide support to patient and family.

Neutropenia

Neutropenia is an abnormally low absolute neutrophil count.

Pathophysiology
- Neutropenia is caused by problems with neutrophil production and/or problems with neutrophil distribution due to infection, treatment, or drugs:
    - *Decreased production of neutrophils* due to aplastic anemia, medications or toxins, metastatic cancer, lymphoma or leukemia, myelodysolastic syndrome, chemotherapy, or radiation.
    - *Increased destruction of neutrophils* (medication induced), due to immunologic disease (e.g., systemic lupus erythematosus), viral disease (e.g., infectious hepatitis, mononucleosis), or bacterial infection.
    - Interruption of neutrophil production or neutrophil distribution → decrease in neutrophil count.

Clinical Presentation
When a patient is neutropenic, the following usual signs of infection may not be present because of the lack of sufficient number of neutrophils needed to produce common infectious signs:
- Fever
- Shaking chills
- Sore throat
- Cough
- SOB
- Nasal congestion
- Diarrhea or loose stools
- Burning during urination
- Unusual redness
- Swelling warmth

Diagnostic Tests
- Blood cultures
- CBC

- Basic metabolic panel (BMP)
- Kidney and liver functions
- Urinalysis and urine culture
- Site-specific cultures, such as stool, skin, and vascular access devices
- Chest x-ray

Management
- Treat with broad-spectrum antibiotics until an organism is identified.
- Check temperature every 4 hours.
- Monitor for signs of infection.
- Assess and monitor CBC with differential.
- Discontinue any medications that could be the cause.
- Educate patient's family members to avoiding visiting if they have cold or flu-like symptoms.
- Maintain good hand washing procedures.

Coagulopathy

Abnormalities in blood coagulation may comprise a large number of disorders, including deficiency (or single-factor) abnormalities and acquired forms associated with multiple coagulation abnormalities. The disorders are discussed here.

Vitamin K Deficiency
Vitamin K deficiency occurs when stores of this vitamin are deficient or abnormal, causing inhibition of normal coagulation.

Pathophysiology
- Prothrombin; factors VII, IX, and X (FVII, FIX, and FX); and proteins C and S are synthesized by the liver through a process that depends on vitamin K.
- Vitamin K deficiency → synthesized hypofunctional by-products → inhibition of normal coagulation. These by-products do not bind to cellular phospholipid surfaces and therefore do not participate in cell-associated coagulation reactions. Coumadin produces a similar coagulation abnormality that antagonizes the action of vitamin K.
- Because the vitamin K is fat soluble, the absorption from the GI tract is decreased in biliary obstruction and in fat malabsorption syndromes.

- Antibiotics that inhibit gut flora decrease amount of vitamin K ordinarily supplied by these organisms.

Clinical Presentation
- Epistaxis and/or bleeding from puncture sites or invasive lines, wounds
- Prolonged PT and elevated international normalized ratio (INR)

Diagnostic Tests
- PT (most sensitive early indicator)

Management
- Administer FFP (treatment of choice for acute hemorrhage or to reverse for a procedure).
- Administer vitamin K (1–10 mg x 3 days).
- Continue to monitor PT.
- Assess for bleeding.
- Provide emotional support to patient and family.

Liver Disease
Coagulation disorder caused by liver disease is multifactoral and involves decreased synthesis of coagulation proteins, decreased clearance of FDPs, and increased fibrinolysis.

Pathophysiology
- In cirrhosis, FVII and protein C are the first to fall → a low FVII level, resulting in a prolonged PT. The remaining vitamin K dependent factors decrease → prolonged aPTT. The fibrinogen level is usually maintained until end-stage disease. Because of impaired synthetic function → factors and fibrinogen may be functionally abnormal.
- In acute toxic or infectious hepatitis, impairment of coagulation correlates with the severity of cell damage.

Unlike the situation with other types of coagulopathy → coagulation factors and fibrinogen may be dysfunctional → because of abnormal hepatic synthetic function platelets may be dysfunctional by circulating FDPs that the liver fails to clear.

Clinical Presentation
- Bleeding
- Prolonged PT, activated PTT (aPTT)
- Elevated FDPs
- Low platelet count

Diagnostic Tests
- PT/PTT
- D-dimer
- Fibrin degradation/split products
- CBC
- Liver function tests

Management
- Administer FFP.
- Administer platelets.
- Administer desmopressin acetate (DDAVP) at 0.3 mcg/kg over 20 minutes (may improve platelet function).

Massive Transfusion

Coagulopathy can be caused by massive transfusion when the replacement of 1 or more blood volumes occurs in a 24-hour period (1 blood volume in a 70-kg adult is about a 5-L blood loss or transfusion volume of 10 units of packed red blood cells [PRBCs]). Common complications of massive transfusion are dilutional coagulopathy, DIC and fibrinolysis, hypothermia, citrate toxicity, hypokalemia, hyperkalemia, and infection.

Pathophysiology

Dilutional thrombocytopenia is the most common cause of bleeding after massive transfusion. If ongoing blood loss is replaced with only PRBCs → fall in platelet count → splenic pool mobilizing and counteracting loss during hemorrhage. If patient's count was high prior to transfusion → remainder may be adequate to prevent bleeding. If pretransfusion count was low or normal → the count may be 50,000–100,000 per microliter → bleeding. Repletion of platelets → enhanced function of the coagulation factors and platelet plug formation. Platelets provide the surface on which many of the factors are activated and fibrin strands are formed.

Clinical Presentation
- Bleeding from areas other than the area of hemorrhage
- Low platelet count
- Prolonged PT, aPTT, and thrombin time
- Decreased fibrinogen

Diagnostic Tests
- PT/PTT
- CBC

HEMA/
ONCO

- D-dimer
- Fibrin degradation/split products

Management
- Administer platelets.
- Administer cryoprecipitate.
- Replace electrolytes as needed.
- Provide support to patient and family members.

For disseminated intravascular coagulation and heparin-induced thrombocytopenia, see pages 159 to 162.

Oncologic Emergencies

Oncologic emergencies are complications or conditions of cancer and/or its treatments requiring urgent or emergent interventions to avoid life-threatening situations.

Sepsis

Sepsis is a condition in which organisms enter into the blood stream, causing activation of the host inflammation defense mechanism → release of cytokines and the activation of plasma protein cascade systems → septic shock → multisystem organ failure. Cancer patients are at an increased risk for sepsis due to ↓ WBC and poor immune systems.

Clinical Presentation
- ↑ WBC
- Fever
- Hypotension
- Tachycardia
- Lethargy
- Agitation and confusion

Diagnostic Tests
- Blood cultures
- Urine cultures and urinalysis
- CBC with differential
- PT/PTT

Management

- Administer broad-spectrum antibiotics until organism identified.
- Support BP with vasopressors, such as vasopressin, Levophed, and dopamine.
- Administer IV fluids.
- Provide emotional support to patient and family members.

Disseminated Intravascular Coagulation

See DIC as previously mentioned on pages 159 to 160.

Syndrome of Inappropriate Antidiuretic Hormone (SIADH)

SIADH is caused by malignant tumors that produce or secrete ADH or tumors that stimulate the brain to make and secrete ADH. SIADH can also be caused by medications frequently used by cancer patients (e.g., morphine, cyclophosphamide). In SIADH, an excessive amount of water is reabsorbed by the kidney → ↑ in excessive fluid in circulation → hyponatremia and fluid retention.

Clinical Presentation
- Weakness
- Muscle cramps
- Loss of appetite
- Fatigue
- Hyponatremia (115–120 mEq/L)
- Weight gain (water weight)
- Nervous system changes
- Personality changes
- Confusion
- Extreme muscle weakness
- If Na^+ <110, may cause possible seizures, coma, and death (if Na^+ <110)

Diagnostic Tests
- Urine electrolytes
- Urinalysis
- BMP (watch Na^+ levels closely)

HEMA/ONCO

Management

■ Restrict fluids.
■ Increase Na$^+$ intake.
■ Drug therapy includes demeclocycline (an antibiotic taken orally that works in opposition to ADH).
■ Radiation or chemotherapy may be given to reduce tumor progression causing SIADH → to normal ADH production.

Spinal Cord Compression

Compression of the spinal cord is caused by a tumor that directly enters the spinal cord or by vertebrae collapsing due to deterioration of the bone secondary to a tumor. The compression site can be from a primary tumor but is usually due to metastases from the lung, prostate, breast, or colon.

Clinical Presentation

■ Back pain
■ Numbness
■ Tingling
■ Loss of urethral, vaginal, and rectal sensation
■ Muscle weakness (neurologic deficits are later signs)
■ Paralysis (usually permanent)

Diagnostic Tests

■ CT scan of torso
■ MRI of spine

Management

■ Provide early recognition and treatment.
■ Perform comprehensive neurologic examination.
■ Administer high-dose corticosteroids to reduce swelling and relieve symptoms.
■ Administer high-dose radiation to reduce tumor size and relieve symptoms.
■ Surgery may be indicated in order to remove the tumor.
■ Apply external neck or back braces.

Hypercalcemia

Cancer in the bone → bone releasing calcium into bloodstream → ↑ serum calcium levels. Cancer in other parts of the body (especially lung, head and neck, kidney, or lymph nodes) → secretion of parathyroid hormone by the tumor → release of calcium by the bone → ↑ serum calcium levels. Decreased mobility and dehydration worsen hypercalcemia.

Clinical Presentation
- Fatigue
- Loss of appetite
- Nausea and vomiting
- Constipation
- Polyuria (early sign)
- Severe muscle weakness
- Loss of deep-tendon reflexes
- Paralytic ileus
- More severe changes: dehydration, ECG changes

Diagnostic Tests
- Parathyroid hormone levels
- BMP q6h (every 6 hours)
- Ionized calcium levels

Management
- Provide oral hydration.
- Provide IV hydration with normal saline.
- Administer medications to decrease calcium levels temporarily.
- Administer glucocorticoids.
- Administer calcitonin.
- Administer diphosphonate.
- Administer mithramycin.
- Dialysis may be indicated to decrease serum calcium levels in life-threatening situations or in those with renal impairment.

Superior Vena Cava Syndrome

SVC syndrome occurs when the superior vena cava is compressed or obstructed by tumor growth → painful life-threatening emergency, most often seen in lymphomas and lung cancer. SVC results in blockage of blood flow in the venous system of the chest, neck, and upper trunk.

Clinical Presentation
Early Symptoms
- Edema of the face, especially around the eyes, when patient arises from night's sleep
- Tightness of shirt or collar (Stoke's sign) as compression worsens
- Edema in arms and hands, dyspnea, erythema of upper body, and epistaxis

Late Symptoms
- Hemorrhage
- Cyanosis
- Mental status changes
- Decreased cardiac output → hypotension
- Death (if compression not relieved)

Diagnostic Tests
- CT of chest
- ECG

Management
- Provide high-dose radiation to the mediastinal area (provides temporary relief).
- Provide interventional radiology may place a metal stent in the vena cava to relieve swelling.
- Follow-up angioplasty may be needed to keep the stent open longer.
- Surgery is rarely performed, because the tumor may have caused such an increase in intrathoracic pressure that closing the chest post-operatively would be impossible.
- Best treatment results occur in the early stages of SVC syndrome.

Tumor Lysis Syndrome

TLS occurs when large numbers of tumor cells are destroyed rapidly → the release of intracellular contents (potassium and purines) into the bloodstream faster than the body can eliminate them → tissue damage and death if severe or untreated ↑ potassium levels → severe hyperkalemia → severe cardiac dysfunction. An ↑ in purines (converted in the liver to uric acid) released into bloodstream → hyperuricemia → precipitation of these crystals in the kidney → sludge in the tubules → blockage → acute renal failure. TLS is most often seen in patients receiving chemotherapy or radiation for the cancers highly responsive to this treatment, including leukemia, lymphoma, small cell lung carcinoma, and multiple myeloma. This oncologic emergency is a positive sign the treatment is working.

Diagnostic Tests
- CMP
- CBC
- ECG
- Ultrasound of kidneys
- Uric acid level

Management
- Provide IV hydration, which ↓ serum K^+ level and ↑ kidney filtration rate.
- Instruct patient to drink at least 3–5 L of fluid the day before, the day of, and 3 days after treatment (especially in patient with tumors highly sensitive to treatment, as mentioned earlier).
- Ensure that some fluids are alkaline (Na^+).
- Health teach importance of consistent fluid intake over 24 hours (help patient draw up a schedule).
- Health teach importance of taking antiemetics after treatment to prevent nausea and vomiting, which would hinder fluid intake.
- Administer diuretics, especially osmotic types, to increase urine flow.
  *Use with caution as diuretics may cause dehydration.
- Administer medications that increase secretion of purines: allupurinol (Zyloprim), rasburicase (Elitek).
- Administer medications to decrease hyperkalemia: sodium polystyrene sulfonate (Kayexalate), either orally or rectally by enema.

- Administer IV infusion containing dextrose and insulin if hyperglycemic.
- Initiate dialysis as needed.

Leukemia

Leukemia is the uncontrolled neoplastic reproduction of white blood cells. Causes include significant bone marrow damage that can result from radiation or chemicals.

Pathophysiology
Myeloid Leukemia
- **Acute:** Malignant alterations in hematopoietic stem cells. Risk factors include advanced age, therapeutic radiation, supportive care patients, smoking, and exposure to chemicals. It is the more common form of myeloid leukemia.
- **Chronic:** Uncontrolled mutation of myeloid cells. This disease is rare in children, and risk increases with age. There is an increased incidence of this type of leukemia with radiation exposure.

Lymphocytic Leukemia
- **Acute:** Large amount of bone marrow stem cells develop into lymphocytes. Most prevalent in young children.
- **Chronic:** Only leukemia not related to radiation or chemicals. B lymphocytes do not go through apoptosis → excessive cells in bone marrow and blood → enlarged nodes → hepatomegaly and splenomegaly → anemia and thrombocytopenia. There is a slight genetic predisposition with this type of leukemia.

Clinical Presentation
Acute Myeloid Leukemia
- Fatigue
- Bruising or bleeding
- Fever
- Infection
- Pain from enlargement of liver and spleen
- Gum hyperplasia
- Bone pain

Chronic Myeloid Leukemia
- Remain asymptomatic in many patients for long periods of time
- Malaise
- Loss of appetite
- Weight loss
- Spleen tenderness and enlargement

Acute Lymphocytic Leukemia
- Reduced leukocytes, erythrocytes, and platelets
- Pain from bone, liver, or spleen
- Headache
- Vomiting

Chronic Lymphocytic Leukemia
- Asymptomatic in many cases
- Elevated WBC
- Enlarged lymph nodes and spleen
- Possible development of B-symptoms: fever, night sweats, weight loss, bacterial infections, and viral infections

Diagnostic Tests
- CBC

Management
- Perform daily assessment of body systems and monitor for anemia and infections.
- Monitor CBC closely.
- Maintain bleeding precautions.
- Provide nutritional support.
- Provide meticulous oral hygiene.
- Provide perirectal hygiene.
- Apply mask to patient when out of room.
- Assess anxiety level.
- Monitor intake and output, and assess hydration status.
- Administer analgesic and antipyretics; provide comfort measures as needed.
- Provide emotional support to patient and family members.

Bone Marrow Transplantation

Bone marrow transplantation is the aspiration of marrow from the posterior iliac crest of a marrow donor under regional or general anesthesia and the IV transfusion of the marrow into a donor-matched recipient.

Procedure
Before being ready to receive the transplant, the patient must:

- Undergo high-dose chemotherapy with or without total body irradiation in an effort to treat the underlying disease and overcome rejection.
- Be treated with immunosuppressive drugs to decrease the risk of rejection. T Factors influencing the outcome of bone marrow transplantation include:
  - Disease status at transplantation
  - Type of donor
  - Recipient's age
  - Comorbid medical conditions

Early-Stage Complications
The time of greatest risk is between 0 and 100 days.

- Rejection
- Mucositis, pain issues secondary to oral ulcerations and reactive herpes virus; oral nutritional deficits secondary to oral pain
- Hemorrhage, caused by chronic thrombocytopenia and tissue injury; can be life threatening, but rare
- Common minor bleeding, such as petechiae, epitaxis, or GI or GU bleeding (not life threatening, but worrisome to patients)
- Infections
  - Bacterial; usually gram-positive, but can be gram-negative
  - Fungal
  - Viral; can be life threatening to these patients
- Acute graft-versus-host disease: One of the most serious and challenging complications; caused by immunologically competent donor-derived T cells that react with recipient tissue antigens
- Venoocclusive disease of the liver: One of the most feared complications; signs and symptoms include unexplained weight gain, jaundice, abdominal pain, and ascites

■ Pulmonary complications: A common problem; causes of lung injury or pneumonitis can be infection, chemical, bleeding, or idiopathic.

Management

■ Provide emotional support to patient and family.
■ Perform good hand washing and aseptic technique.
■ Use reverse isolation procedures.
■ Monitor CBC and BMP laboratory tests frequently.
■ Provide frequent oral care.
■ Assess for signs and symptoms of bleeding.
■ Monitor vital signs every 4 hours or more frequently if needed.
■ Administer immunosuppressive drugs as ordered.
■ Consider IV or enteral nutritional support.

Diabetic Ketoacidosis

DKA is a life-threatening metabolic complication caused by an absence or inadequate amount of insulin. Affecting mostly type 1 diabetics, it is marked by three concurrent abnormalities: hyperglycemia, dehydration and electrolyte loss, and metabolic acidosis.

Pathophysiology

DKA can be initiated by trauma or conditions such as new-onset diabetes, heart failure, or stress. The body under stress → decrease in the amount of insulin → reduction of glucose entering cells and increased glucose production by the liver → hyperglycemia → liver attempting to get rid of excess glucose by excreting glucose with water, Na^+ and K^+ → polyuria → dehydration.

DKA can also be caused by a lack of insulin → increased breakdown of fat → increased fatty acid and glycerol → fatty acids converted into ketones → acidosis → increasing respiratory rate and abdominal pain, and acetone breath.

Clinical Presentation

- Hyperglycemia
- Polyuria
- Dehydration
- Weakness
- Headache
- Polydipsia
- Acetone or fruity breath
- Poor appetite
- Nausea and vomiting
- Abdominal pain, usually generalized or epigastric
- Rigid abdomen and irregular bowel sounds
- Kussmaul's respirations
- Hypothermia
- Tachycardia
- Hypotension
- Glycosuria

- Ketones in blood and urine
- Metabolic acidosis: pH <7.3, bicarbonate <15 mmol/L, blood glucose >14 mmol/L, and ketonuria

Diagnostic Tests

- Electrocardiogram
- Chest x-ray
- Urinalysis (note presence of ketones)
- CBC
- Serum electrolytes, glucose and ketone levels, and blood urea nitrogen
- Urine, sputum, and wound and blood cultures
- Arterial blood gases (ABGs) and anion gap (8–16 mEq/L or 8–16 mmol/L normal)
- Plasma osmolarity
- Cardiac enzymes
- Amylase and lipase levels

Note: Serum and urine should be negative for ketones.

Management

- Provide airway support.
- Administer O_2 (3–6 L via nasal cannula).
- Monitor respiratory rate and rhythm and blood pH.
- Monitor vital signs.
- Assess for changes in mental status.
- Assess for signs of hypokalemia.
- Monitor serum glucose and ketone levels.
- Provide insulin replacement (insulin drip).
- Provide electrolyte replacement.
- Provide fluid resuscitation and monitor intake and output.

Diabetes Insipidus

DI is a disease manifested by the excretion of a large volume of urine caused by ineffective production of antidiuretic hormone (ADH) at the posterior pituitary.

Pathophysiology

The four types of DI include:
■ Central DI
  ■ No ADH secretion
  ■ Cause can be congenital or idiopathic:
    • Tumors in the central nervous system
    • Cerebrovascular disease or trauma
    • Infection
    • Granulomas
    • Pregnancy
    • Brain death
■ Nephrogenic DI
  ■ Secretion of ADH but no stimulation to the nephron's collecting tubules
  ■ Cause can be congenital or idiopathic:
    • Obstruction that hinders normal urine excretion
    • Chronic tubulointerstitial disease
    • Medications
    • Electrolyte imbalance
■ Dipsogenic DI
  ■ Caused by a defect or damage to the thirst mechanism in the hypothalamus
  ■ Results in an abnormal increase in thirst with an increased fluid intake that suppresses ADH secretion and increases urine output
■ Gestational DI
  ■ Occurs only during pregnancy

Clinical Presentation

■ Large volume of very diluted urine with a low specific gravity (volume does not decrease even with restricted fluids)
■ Extreme thirst, especially for cold water and sometimes ice or ice water
■ Craving for fluid
■ Dehydration
■ Symptoms of hypovolemic shock: Changes in level of consciousness (LOC), tachycardia, tachypnea, and hypotension

Diagnostic Tests

- Fluid deprivation test
- Desmopressin stimulation
- ADH test
- Plasma and urine osmolarity
- Serum chemistries and electrolytes
- Urinalysis
- CT scan of head to detect cranial lesions

Management

- Administer desmopressin; ineffective in nephrogenic DI.
- Administer hydrochlorothiazide or indomethacin (Indocin) for nephrogenic DI.
- If surgery is needed, provide emotional support to patient and family.
- Assess intake and output.
- Monitor vital signs frequently.
- Administer fluids as needed.

Adrenal Crisis

Acute crisis, also known as acute adrenal insufficiency, is a serious complication of a dysfunctional adrenal gland causing difficulties producing aldosterone and cortisol hormones.

Pathophysiology

Destruction of adrenal cortex → hindered secretion of aldosterone and cortisol → Addison's disease → hypoglycemia and hypovolemic shock.

Causes of adrenal crisis include:

- Recently halted chronic corticosteroid therapy
- Injury to or infection of the adrenal gland
- Chronic adrenal insufficiency
- Bilateral adrenalectomy
- Medications that suppress adrenal hormones
- Medications that enhance steroid metabolism
- Sepsis

Clinical Presentation

- Serious weakness and fatigue
- Hypoglycemia
- Fever
- Vomiting
- Diarrhea
- Altered mental status and confusion
- Hypotension
- Tachycardia
- Dysrhythmias
- Lack of response to vasopressors

Diagnostic Tests

- Cosyntropin (ACTH) stimulation test
- CT scan or ultrasound of the adrenal glands

Management

- Assess vital signs.
- Weigh daily.
- Strictly monitor intake and output.
- Monitor serum glucose levels frequently.
- Administer IV fluids.
- Administer cortisol replacement medications (hydrocortisone IV).
- Insert nasogastric tube if vomiting.
- Reorient and minimize stress.
- Provide small frequent meals and nutritional supplements.

Thyroid Storm

Thyroid storm is a rare life-threatening complication of a severe form of hyperthyroidism that is characterized by high fever, extreme tachycardia, and altered mental status, and is precipitated by stress.

Pathophysiology

Thyrotropin-releasing hormone (TRH) is released from the hypothalamus after exposure to stress → the pituitary gland releasing thyroid-stimulating hormone (TSH) → causes the release of thyroid hormone (T_3 and T_4) from the thyroid gland → T_3 active form of thyroid hormone → increased levels of thyroid hormone leading to hyperthyroidism or thyrotoxicosis → if precipitated by stress (surgery, infection, trauma, DKA, heart failure, pulmonary embolism, toxemia of pregnancy, thyroid hormone ingestion, radioiodine therapy, discontinuation of antithyroid), further increase in serum TH → thyroid storm.

Clinical Presentation

- High fever and hyperthermia
- Severe tachycardia (>200 bpm) with heart failure and shock
- Restlessness and agitation
- Abdominal pain
- Goiter
- Nausea and vomiting
- Nervousness
- Tremor
- Confusion
- Delirium
- Coma

Exaggerated symptoms of hyperthyroidism with disturbances of major systems:

- GI:
  - Weight loss
  - Diarrhea
  - Abdominal pain
- CV:
  - Edema
  - Chest pain
  - Dyspnea
  - Palpitations

Diagnostic Tests

- Serum thyroid panel
- Liver function tests

Management

"Triangle of Treatment":

- Decrease sympathetic outflow (beta blockers: esmolol–drug of choice).
- Decrease production of TH (propylthiouracil [PTU] or methimazole).
- Decrease peripheral conversion of T_4 to T_3 (PTU, beta blockers, and steroids).
- Prevent cardiac collapse.
- Administer humidified O_2.
- Monitor ABGs and provide continuous pulse oximetry monitoring.
- Monitor vital signs frequently.
- Administer IV fluids containing dextrose to replace liver glycogen.
- Give beta blockers; if contraindicated, give calcium channel blockers to prevent excessive hyperthermia.
- Give acetaminophen; salicylates are contraindicated.
- Monitor intake and output.

Syndrome of Inappropriate Antidiuretic Hormone

SIADH is the continuous production of ADH from the pituitary gland despite low osmolarity. It is frequently manifested by hyponatremia.

Pathophysiology

Malignant tumors, disorders of CNS and medications → increased secretion of ADH → hyponatremia → increased water retention → stimulation of renin-angiotensin system → increased excretion of sodium in urine.

Clinical Presentation

- Concentrated urine
- Water retention
- Lethargy
- Dilutional hyponatremia
- Signs and symptoms of hyponatremia:
  - Poor skin turgor and dry mucosa
  - Headache
  - Decreased saliva
  - Orthostatic hypotension
  - Anorexia, nausea, and vomiting
  - Abdominal cramps
  - Irritability, confusion, and disorientation
  - Seizures

Diagnostic Tests

- Comprehensive metabolic panel
- Urine Na$^+$ and electrolytes
- Serum and urine osmolarity
- Ultrasound of kidneys
- CT scan of head

Management

- Monitor intake and output.
- Weigh daily.
- Monitor for CNS changes.
- Assess for edema of extremities.
- Institute fluid restrictions.
- Closely monitor electrolytes.
- Administer demeclocycline (Declomycin, Declostatin, Ledermycin) to treat hyponatremia by inhibiting the action of ADH.
- Administer conivaptan (Vaprisol) to treat hyponatremia.
- Provide emotional support.

Shock

The 3 types of shock include:

- **Hypovolemic shock:** Due to decreased circulating or intravascular volume
- **Cardiogenic shock:** Due to the inability of the heart to pump effectively
- **Distributive shock:** Due to maldistribution of circulating blood volume. Examples include:
  - Septic shock (caused by an infectious process)
  - Anaphylactic shock (a hypersensitivity reaction)
  - Neurogenic shock (due to alterations in vascular smooth muscle tone)

Pathophysiology

The pathophysiology of shock is complex and not fully understood.

- Blood volume displaced in the vasculature → ↓ cardiac output (CO) → ↓ tissue perfusion → ↑ HR and contractility with shunting of blood to the vital organs (brain).
- Renin-angiotensin response → angiotensin II (vasoconstriction) → release of aldosterone and antidiuretic hormone → Na^+ and H_2O retention → ↑ preload.
- Stimulation of the anterior pituitary gland → secretion of adrenocorticotropic hormone → stimulation of adrenal cortex → release of glucocorticoids → ↑ blood glucose.
- Stimulation of the adrenal medulla → release of epinephrine and norepinephrine → cell metabolism changes from aerobic to anaerobic → lactic acidosis.
- Cardiac hypoperfusion → ventricular failure.
- Cerebral hypoperfusion → failure of sympathetic nervous system, cardiac and respiratory depression, and thermoregulatory failure.
- Respiratory depression → ↑ pulmonary capillary membrane permeability → pulmonary vasoconstriction, → acute respiratory failure, and acute respiratory distress syndrome (ARDS).
- Renal hypoperfusion → acute tubular necrosis → acute renal failure.
- GI hypoperfusion → failure of GI organs.
- Multiple organ dysfunction syndrome (MODS): the failure of 2 or more body systems → death.

Clinical Presentation

- Systolic BP <90 mm Hg
- $\uparrow$ HR, narrowing of pulse pressure, dysrhythmias, absent peripheral pulses
- Delayed capillary refill and flat jugular veins
- Altered mental status, confusion, altered level of consciousness (LOC) $\rightarrow$ lethargy and unconsciousness
- Hypoxemia and respiratory alkalosis initially due to $\uparrow$ respiratory rate (RR) and $\uparrow$ depth of respirations $\rightarrow$ respiratory distress $\rightarrow$ respiratory failure $\rightarrow$ respiratory and metabolic acidosis
- Oliguria progressing to anuria, and $\uparrow$ urine osmolality and specific gravity
- $\uparrow$ blood urea nitrogen (BUN) and creatinine
- Pale and cool skin progressing to ashen, cold-clammy to cyanotic, mottled, and diaphoretic skin

Diagnostic Tests

- Serum chemistries, including electrolytes, BUN, and creatinine
- CBC and coagulation profile
- Arterial blood gases (ABGs) or pulse oximetry
- Cardiac output studies $\rightarrow$ $\downarrow$ cardiac index (CI), $\downarrow$ cardiac output, $\downarrow$ preload, $\downarrow$ right atrial pressure (RAP), $\uparrow$ afterload, and $\uparrow$ systemic vascular resistance
- Serum lactate
- Urinalysis with specific gravity, osmolarity, and urine electrolytes
- Electrocardiogram (ECG)

Management

- Monitor vital signs and hemodynamics via arterial line and pulmonary artery catheter.
- Institute cardiac monitoring for dysrhythmias.
- Assess respiratory status and ABGs or pulse oximetry.
- Administer O_2 via cannula, mask, or mechanical ventilation. Assess for signs of hypoxia.
- Note skin color and temperature. Control fever.

- Assess neurological status and LOC.
- Administer IV fluids, colloids (.9NS, LR), and crystalloids.
- Insert Foley catheter. Monitor intake and output.
- Assess fluid and electrolyte balance.
- Administer IV vasopressors as indicated by hemodynamic parameters.
- Administer IV vasodilators and diuretic to ↓ preload or afterload.
- Administer sympathomimetics and digoxin to ↑ contractility.
- Administer antiarrhythmics if cardiac dysrhythmias present.
- Provide nutritional support, either enterally or parenterally.
- Institute intra-aortic balloon pump counterpulsation for cardiogenic shock or ventricular assist device.
- Monitor serum lactic acid level. Administer sodium bicarbonate (not recommended in the treatment of shock-related lactic acidosis).
- Provide stress ulcer and deep vein thrombosis (DVT) prophylaxis per institution policy and protocols.
- Provide analgesics for pain. Sedate as necessary.
- Provide emotional support to patient and family. Relieve anxiety.

Medications

Sympathomimetics are administered to improve contractility, ↑ SV, and ↑ CO:

- Dobutamine (Dobutrex)
- Dopamine (Intropin)
- Inamrinone (Amrinone)
- Milrinone (Primacor)
- Epinephrine (Adrenalin)

Vasodilators are administered to ↓ preload and afterload, and to ↓ O_2 demand on the heart:

- Nitroglycerine (Tridil)
- Nitroprusside (Nipride)

Vasoconstrictors are administered to ↑ BP:

- Norepinephrine (Levophed)
- Phenylephrine (Neo-synephrine)

Caution must be used in titrating medications to the patient's hemodynamic response.

Sepsis

In sepsis, microorganisms invade the body, resulting in a systemic inflammatory response syndrome (SIRS) that may lead to septic shock, multiple organ dysfunction syndrome (MODS), and eventually death. Causes are gram (+) and gram (–) aerobes, anaerobes, fungi, and viruses.

Pathophysiology

Sepsis is a condition in which organisms enter into the bloodstream, causing activation of the host inflammation defense mechanism → release of cytokines and the activation of plasma protein cascade systems → septic shock → multisystem organ failure. Cancer patients are at an increased risk for sepsis due to ↓ WBC and poor immune systems.

Clinical Presentation

- T >38°C (100.4°F) or <36°C (96.8°F)
- HR >90 bpm
- RR >20 bpm or partial pressure of arterial carbon dioxide ($PaCO_2$) <32 mm Hg
- WBC >12,000/mm^3, <4,000/mm^3, or >10% immature (band) forms

The presence of 2 or more of the above symptoms indicates SIRS.

- Fever and chills
- Fatigue and malaise
- Warm and pink skin, progressing to cold, clammy, and mottled skin
- Hypotension or normal BP
- Widening pulse pressure
- ↓ RAP and left ventricular stroke work index
- Partial arterial oxygen tension (PaO_2)/fractional concentration of oxygen in inspired gas (FIO_2) ratio <300
- ↑ lactate levels and lactic acidosis
- Decreased urine output progressing to oliguria
- Acute changes in mental status, such as anxiety, apprehension, delirium, disorientation, confusion, combativeness, agitation, lethargy, or coma

- Increased RR, SOB, crackles, hypoxemia progressing to pulmonary edema, acute lung injury, hypoxemia, and respiratory failure
- Nausea, vomiting, jaundice, ↓ GI motility, and ileus
- Changes in carbohydrate, fat, and glucose metabolism
- Signs of thrombocytopenia and coagulopathies (possibly progressing to disseminated intravascular coagulation)
- Possible development of signs of septic shock

Diagnostic Tests

- CBC with differential (↑ or ↓ WBC)
- Serum chemistries, bilirubin, serum lactate (increased), liver function tests (abnormal), and protein C (decreased)
- Insulin resistance with elevated blood glucose
- ABGs (hypoxemia, lactic acidosis)
- Urine, sputum, wound, and blood cultures
- Activated partial thromboplastin time (increased), international normalized ratio (increased), and D-dimer (increased)

Management

Management is dependent on degree of sepsis and whether or not septic shock is present.

Sepsis Resuscitation Bundle

Within 6 hours of diagnosis of severe sepsis:

- Measure serum lactate.
- Obtain blood cultures prior to antibiotic administration.
- Administer broad-spectrum antibiotic within 3 hours of ED admission and within 1 hour of non-ED admission.
- If hypotension is present and/or serum lactate is >4 mmol/L, deliver an initial minimum of 20 mL/kg of crystalloid or equivalent and administer vasopressors for hypotension not responding to fluid resuscitation to maintain mean arterial pressure (MAP) at >65 mm Hg.
- In the case of persistent hypertension and/or elevated lactate levels, achieve a central venous pressure (CVP) of ≥8 mm Hg, and a central venous oxygen saturation of ≥70% or a mixed venous oxygen saturation of ≥65%.

Sepsis Management Bundle

Within 24 hours of presentation with severe sepsis or septic shock:

- Administer low-dose steroids for septic shock.
- Administer drotrecogin alpha (activated).
- Maintain glucose control at $\geq$70 but <150 mg/dL.
- Maintain a median inspiratory plateau pressure of <30 cm H_2O for mechanically ventilated patients.

Other Nursing Care

- Assess vital signs and consider arterial line placement. Monitor mean arterial pressure and maintain at $\geq$65 mm Hg.
- Support BP by administering vasopressors (e.g., vasopressin, Levophed, dopamine).
- Assess hemodynamic status. Consider pulmonary artery catheter placement. Maintain CVP at 8–12 mm Hg.
- Assess respiratory status.
- Monitor ABGs and note $\downarrow$ pH, $\downarrow$ PaO_2, and $\uparrow$ $PaCO_2$.
- Administer O_2 via nasal cannula, mask, or mechanical ventilation. Use minimum positive end-respiratory pressure to achieve tidal volume and end-inspiratory plateau pressure goals.
- Position patient to promote optimal O_2 exchange. Reposition every 2 hours.
- Institute skin care protocols.
- Keep head of bed (HOB) elevated 45°.
- Institute ventilator-associated pneumonia precautions if patient is on mechanical ventilation.
- Treat fever if present.
- Assess neurologic status for changes in mentation.
- Insert Foley catheter and monitor intake and output. Maintain urine output at $\geq$0.5 mL/kg/hr.
- Administer IV colloids and crystalloids, and fluid challenge as necessary. Assess fluid and electrolyte balance.
- Assess nutritional status. Provide enteral feeding or total parenteral nutrition (TPN) and lipids.
- Perform cortisol stimulation test. Start continuous low-dose steroid infusion.

- Administer antibiotics within 1 hour of sepsis diagnosis, and re-evaluate 48–72 hours afterward.
- Administer vasopressors and inotropes. Consider Vasopressin for refractory shock.
- Monitor blood glucose levels and maintain tight glucose control at 80–110 mg/dL. Consider insulin infusion.
- Administer platelets if platelet count is <5,000/mm^3.
- Institute stress ulcer and DVT prophylaxis.
- Prevent nosocomial infections.
- Sedate patient as necessary.
- Administer drotrecogin alfa (Xigris): An anticoagulant, profibrinolytic, anti-inflammatory agent.

Systemic Inflammatory Response Syndrome

SIRS is a widespread inflammation that may progress to acute lung injury, acute renal failure, MODS, and eventually death.

SIRS is diagnosed if one or more of the following signs are present:

- T >38°C (100.4°F) or <36°C (96.8°F)
- HR >90 bpm
- Tachypnea with RR >20 bpm or PaCO$_2$ <32 mm Hg
- WBC count >12,000 cells/mm^3 or <4,000 cells/mm^3, or >10% immature neutrophils

Signs, symptoms, and management are similar to those for sepsis, severe sepsis, and septic shock.

Multiple Organ Dysfunction Syndrome

MODS is defined as the physiologic failure of two or more separate organ systems. With MODS, homeostasis can not be maintained without specific interventions due to the body's inability to sufficiently activate its own defense mechanisms.

Those at high risk for developing MODS include patients with:

- Multiple trauma
- Massive infection or sepsis
- Hemorrhage or shock

- Surgical complications
- Acute pancreatitis
- Burns, extensive tissue damage, and/or necrotic tissue
- Aspiration
- Multiple blood transfusions
- Inadequate fluid resuscitation

Signs, symptoms, and management are similar to those for sepsis, severe sepsis, and septic shock. The need for dialysis is an early warning sign of MODS.

Trauma

Pathophysiology

- **Blunt trauma:** Due to motor vehicle crashes (MVCs), falls, blows, explosions, contact sports, and blunt force injuries, such as from a baseball bat.
  - Estimating the amount of force a person sustains in an MVC = person's weight $\times$ miles per hour of speed.
  - During an MVC, the body stops but the tissues and organs continue to move forward and then backward (acceleration-deceleration force).
- **Penetrating trauma:** Due to gunshot wounds, stabbings, and firearms or implement (missile, shrapnel) injuries.
  - There is direct damage to internal structures, with damage occurring along the path of penetration.
  - Penetrating trauma usually requires surgery.
- **Traumatic brain injury (TBI):** Results from a skull fracture, concussion, contusion, cerebral hematoma, and diffuse axonal injury.
- **Chest or thoracic injuries:** Result from either blunt trauma or a penetrating injury.
  - Common injuries include rib fractures, flail chest, ruptured diaphragm, aortic disruption, pulmonary contusion, tension or open pneumothorax, hemothorax, penetrating or blunt cardiac injuries, and cardiac tamponade.
- **Abdominal injuries:** Caused by blunt trauma or penetrating injury.
  - Common injuries include liver and spleen damage, renal trauma, bladder trauma, and pelvic fractures.

- **Musculoskeletal injuries:** Include spinal cord injury, fracture, dislocation, amputation, and tissue trauma.
  - Fat embolism may occur secondary to fractures of the long bones.

Diagnostic Tests

- CBC
- Serum chemistry panel, including electrolytes, glucose, BUN, and
  creatinine
- Liver function tests
- Serum amylase if pancreatic injury suspected or GI perforation is
  present
- Serum lactate level
- Prothrombin time (PT) and PTT
- Urinalysis
- ABGs or pulse oximetry
- ECG
- Type and crossmatch for possible blood transfusion
- Drug and alcohol toxicology screens
- Pregnancy test for females of childbearing age
- X-rays specific to injury (e.g., chest, abdomen and pelvis, extremity)
- CT scan of the abdomen (ultrasound if indicated)
- Diagnostic peritoneal lavage if internal abdominal bleeding suspected
- Rectal or vaginal exam if indicated

Management

Management is dependent on type of trauma.

- Maintain patent airway. Assess respiratory status for signs of trauma,
  tachypnea, accessory muscle use, tracheal shift, stridor, hyperreso-
  nance, dullness to percussion, rate depth, and symmetry.
- Monitor ABGs or pulse oximetry.
- Observe for respiratory distress.
- Assess chest wall integrity for flail chest or pneumothorax.
- Administer O_2 via nasal cannula, mask, or mechanical ventilation. Use
  oropharyngeal or nasopharyngeal airway or endotracheal tube.
- Insert chest tube if pneumothorax is present.

- Assess for signs of bleeding. Control hemorrhage. Transfuse as needed. Consider autotransfusion of shed blood, autologous blood, unmatched type-specific blood, or type O (universal donor) blood.
- Consider pneumatic antishock garment to control hemorrhage.
- Replace each mL of blood loss with 3 mL of crystalloid (3:1 rule).
- Monitor vital signs frequently, and assess for signs of hypovolemic shock. Maintain BP within acceptable parameters.
- Provide continuous cardiac monitoring.
- Provide peripheral IV access or insert a central venous catheter for IV fluids. Use rapid infuser devices as needed.
- Assess neurological status for confusion and disorientation. Use Glasgow Coma Scale.
- Immobilize the spine and cervical area until assessment is made of spinal cord injury, and head and neck injuries.
- Prevent hypothermia through the use of blankets, warming blankets, or warming lights.
- Insert Foley catheter. Monitor intake and output. Assess fluid and electrolyte balance. Assess urine for bleeding.
- Assess abdomen. Note bowel sounds, guarding, bruising, tenderness, pain, rigidity, and rebound tenderness.
- Perform peritoneal lavage if abdominal injury is present.
- Insert nasogastric tube (NG) tube to prevent gastric distention, decrease risk for aspiration, and assess for GI bleeding.
- Provide nutritional support orally, enterally (gastric, duodenal, or jejunal route), or parenterally (TPN and lipids).
- Note skin color, pallor, bruising, distended neck veins, and edema.
- Inspect for soft tissue injury, deformities, wounds, ecchymosis, and tenderness. Palpate for crepitus and subcutaneous emphysema.
- Administer broad-spectrum antibiotics to prevent and treat infection. Observe for sepsis. Avoid nosocomial infections.
- Provide analgesics for pain. Sedate as necessary.
- Provide DVT and stress ulcer prophylaxis.
- Administer tetanus prophylaxis.

Complications

- Hypermetabolism; occurs 24 to 48 hours after traumatic injury
- Infection and sepsis; SIRS

- Acute respiratory failure or ARDS
- DVT; pulmonary or fat embolism
- Acute renal failure
- Compartment syndrome
- Dilutional coagulopathy
- MODS

Induced or Therapeutic Hypothermia

In order to reduce the damage to brain cells through reduction of the brain's metabolic activity, hypothermia is intentionally induced by bringing the core body temperature down to 32°–34°C (89.6°–93.2°F) Indications for medically induced hypothermia include:

- Ischemic cerebral or spinal injury, including stroke recovery
- Cerebral edema and increased intracranial pressure
- Heart surgery
- Cardiac arrest due to ventricular fibrillation (VF) or ventricular tachycardia; this is most effective within 6 hours of cardiac arrest

Hypothermia may be accomplished by several methods:

- Rapid infusion of ice-cold IV fluids
- NG lavage with ice water
- Evaporative cooling of the external body surface
- External cooling with ice packs or special cooling blankets
- Prevention of shivering and fever

The patient may be rewarmed through the use of:

- Cardiopulmonary bypass
- Warm IV fluid administration
- Warm humidified O_2 administration via ventilator
- Warm peritoneal lavage
- Warming blankets and over-the-bed heaters

Caution should be taken with active core rewarming, because VF can occur as the patient's temperature increases.

Burns

Burns may be thermal, electrical, or chemical.

Type of Burn	Extent of Burn Injury	Description of Burn Injury
First-degree burn or superficial partial-thickness burn	• Epidermis destroyed • Portion of dermis injured	• Red and dry • May be blistered • Blanching with pressure • Little or no edema • Tingling • Supersensitivity • Pain soothed by cooling
Second-degree burn or deep partial-thickness burn	• Epidermis and upper layer of dermis destroyed • Injury to deeper portions of dermis	• Painful wound • Red or pale, mottled • Blistered, edema • Fluid exudate • Hair follicles intact • ↓ blanching with pressure • Sensitive to cold air
Third-degree or full-thickness burn	• Epidermis and dermis destroyed • Underlying tissue may be destroyed	• Pale white, cherry red, brown, or black leathery eschar • Broken skin with fat exposed • Edema • No blanching with pressure • Painless • Hair follicles and sweat glands destroyed

Continued

Type of Burn	Extent of Burn Injury	Description of Burn Injury
Fourth-degree or full-thickness burn	• Skin, fascia, muscle, and bone are irreversibly destroyed.	• Hard, leather-like eschar • No sensation • Charred bones

A cold burn may occur when the skin is in contact with cold bodies, such as snow or cold air, as in cases of frostbite, or is exposed to dry ice or canned air. The treatment is the same for this type of burn.

Pathophysiology

Burns of <25% total body surface area (TBSA) → local response to injury.
Burns of >25% TBSA → local and systemic response to injury.
There are three zones of thermal injury:

- Zone of coagulation where there is irreversible tissue necrosis.
- Zone of stasis surrounding the zone of coagulation.
  - There is ↓ blood flow to the area and vascular damage.
  - Tissue damage may potentially be reversed with adequate care and treatment.
- Zone of hyperemia surrounding the zone of stasis.
  - There is minimal injury to the area and evidence of early recovery.

Burn Stages
The two burn stages are the resuscitative phase and the acute phase.

Resuscitative Phase
- The resuscitative phase begins at the time of injury and continues during the first 48–72 hours, until fluid and protein shifts are stabilized.
- Burn tissue injury occurs → loss of capillary integrity → ↑ permeability of capillary membrane → fluid shifts from the vascular to the interstitial spaces → ↓ CO, ↓ BP, and ↑ HR and peripheral vasoconstriction → ↓ renal blood flow → ↓ renal function → acute renal failure.
- Na^+ and fluid pass through the burn areas → blisters, local edema, and fluid exudate → compartment syndrome.

- K^+ is released from the tissue injury and there is ↓ renal excretion of K^+ → hyperkalemia.
- Lysis of red blood cells (RBCs) occurs → hematuria, myoglobin in the urine, and anemia.
- Coagulation abnormalities occur → prolonged clotting and prothrombin times.
- Metabolic acidosis occurs.
- General tissue hypoperfusion occurs due to ↓ circulating blood volume → burn shock → ↓ BP and tachycardia.
- Hypothermia occurs due to loss of skin barrier → thermoregulation problems.

Acute Phase

- The acute phase of burn injury is characterized by the onset of diuresis. It generally begins approximately 48–72 hours after the burn injury.
- Capillary membrane integrity returns → fluid shifts from interstitial to intravascular space → ↑ in blood volume → diuresis if good renal function exists.
- Fluid overload can occur.
- Hemodilution causes a ↓ in serum electrolytes and hematocrit.
- Na^+ deficit may continue.
- K^+ moves back into the cells → hypokalemia.
- Protein continues to be lost from the wound.

- Calculation of TBSA injured according to the rule of nines:

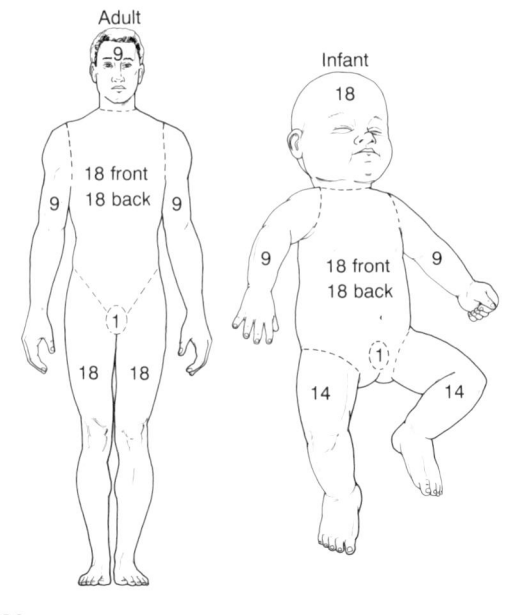

- CBC
- Serum chemistry panel, including electrolytes, glucose, BUN, and creatinine
- Liver function tests
- Serum lactate level
- PT and PTT
- Urinalysis (especially specific gravity, pH, glucose, acetone, protein, and myoglobin)

- ABGs or pulse oximetry, and carboxyhemoglobin (COHgb)
- ECG
- Type and crossmatch for blood
- Drug and alcohol toxicology screens
- Pregnancy test for women of childbearing age
- X-rays specific to injury (e.g., chest, abdomen and pelvis, extremity)
- CT scan of abdomen (ultrasound if indicated)
- Bronchoscopy if inhalation injury is present

Management

Management of burns depends on the location of the burn and the extent of the burn injury.

- Maintain patent airway. Intubate or perform tracheostomy as needed. Administer 100% humidified O_2 by nasal cannula, mask, or mechanical ventilation/continuous positive airway pressure.
- Assess respiratory status. Encourage the use of incentive spirometer, coughing and deep breathing, suctioning, or bronchodilators. Note respiratory distress.
- Monitor ABGs or pulse oximetry for hypoxemia. Monitor COHgb levels.
- Monitor for and prevent pneumonia.
- Immobilize the spine until assessment can be made of injury.
- Irrigate chemical burns immediately.
- Assess TBSA burned and depth of burn injuries.
- Provide analgesics for pain. Maintain good pain control.
- Initiate IV fluid resuscitation to replace fluid and electrolytes:
  - Consensus Formula recommendation is to give 2 mL/kg per percentage burn of lactated Ringer's solution
  - One half of the calculated total is given over the 1st 8 hours postburn injury, and the other half is given over the next 16 hours.
- Provide IV fluid boluses if ↓ BP
- Consider insertion of pulmonary artery catheter to monitor hemodynamics.
- Insert arterial line to monitor BP and obtain blood specimens.
- Palpate peripheral pulses. Use Doppler if necessary.
- Provide continuous ECG monitoring.
- Insert NG tube if burn is >25% of the TBSA. Note GI bleeding.

- Assess GI status, noting bowel sounds, abdominal distention, and nausea. Administer antiemetics if nausea and vomiting present.
- Keep patient NPO initially. Assess nutritional status and provide feedings orally, enterally, or parenterally. Maintain aspiration precautions.
- Insert Foley catheter. Monitor intake and output with goal of 30–50 mL of urine/hr. Note hematuria. Burgundy colored urine is composed of hemochromogen and myoglobin.
- Weigh patient daily. Note height on admission to unit.
- Monitor electrolyte balance.
- Assess neurological status for restlessness, confusion, difficulty concentrating, and changes in LOC.
- Assess warmth, capillary refill time, sensation, and movement of extremities.
- Keep HOB elevated 30°–45°. Elevate burned extremities.
- Provide tetanus prophylaxis.
- Monitor for infection and sepsis. Prevent nosocomial infection. Provide aseptic management of burn areas and invasive lines.
- Provide DVT and stress ulcer prophylaxis.
- Provide active and passive range-of-motion exercises.
- Treat anemia. Consider blood transfusions. Monitor coagulation factors.
- Provide warm environment through the use of clean sheets and blankets, or warm IV fluids.
- Monitor temperature, and prevent chills and shivering.
- Provide psychosocial support to patient and family. Be alert for signs of depression. Provide antianxiety medications.
- In the elderly, balance the risk of hypovolemia and fluid overload.
- In circumferential burns (burn completely surrounds body part), assess need for escharotomy, in which an incision is made through a full-thickness chest wound to decrease constriction, relieve pressure, and restore ventilation (chest) and/or improve blood flow and tissue perfusion.

Wound Care
- Cleanse wound as per protocol.
- Prepare patient for wound debridement (natural, mechanical, or surgical).
- Initiate topical antibacterial therapy:
  - Silver sulfadiazine (Silvadene) 1%
  - Silver nitrate aqueous solution ($AgNO_3$) 0.5%

- Mafenide acetate (Sulfamylon) 5%–10%
- Acticoat (silver-coated dressing)
- Aquacel Ag (silver-coated dressing)
- Silverlon (silver-coated dressing)
- Clotrimazole cream or nystatin (Mycostatin) if fungal infection is present
- Diluted Dakin's solution
- Petroleum-based ointments (bacitracin, gentamycin)
- A vacuum-assisted closure (VAC) device may be used for wound healing along with a variety of dressings.

Patient/Hospital Specific Wound and Dressing Protocol

_____
_____
_____
_____
_____
_____
_____
_____
_____
_____

Wound Grafting

A variety of biological and synthetic skin grafts may be used for wound grafting:

- Hemografts or allografts: Skin from another human, such as a cadaver
- Heterografts or xenografts: Skin from another animal, such as pigskin
- Autografts: Skin from oneself that is transferred from one part of the body to another
- Temporary biosynthetic skin substitutes: Biobrane and TransCyte
- Permanent biosynthetic skin substitutes: Integra and Alloderm

Complications

- Hypovolemia
- Decreased renal function, possibly leading to acute renal failure

- Infection and sepsis
- Paralytic ileus (↓ bowel sounds, distention, and nausea and vomiting)
- Curling's ulcer (stress ulcer or duodenal erosion)
- Metabolic acidosis
- Tissue necrosis
- Hypothermia
- Acute respiratory failure and ARDS
- VAP
- Scarring
- Compromised immunity
- Changes in functional status, appearance, and body image, with associated depression
- Compartment syndrome occurring due to increased pressure in the fascial compartments of an extremity → compression and occlusion of blood vessels and nerves to the extremity. Symptoms include delayed capillary refill, tense skin, progressively diminishing or absent pulse to the extremity, intense pain, paresthesia, and paralysis of the extremity → ischemia and necrosis → loss of limb. Escharotomy is the treatment of choice.
- Abdominal compartment syndrome with symptoms including an increase in intra-abdominal pressure, decreased urine output, and difficulty with ventilation. This condition is treated by laparotomy, trunk escharotomies, and diuretics.

Commonly Used Critical Care Medications

adenosine, **Adenocard**: antidysrhythmic. Uses: SVT, as a diagnostic aid to assess myocardial perfusion defects in CAD. Usual dosages: **IV Bolus** 6 mg, if conversion to NSR does not occur within 1–2 minutes, give 12 mg by rapid **IV Bolus**, may repeat 12–mg dose again in 1–2 min.

alteplase, **Activase**: Thrombolytic enzyme. Uses: Lysis of obstructing thrombi associated with AMI, ischemic conditions requiring thrombolysis (i.e., PE, DVT, unclotting arteriovenous shunts, acute ischemic CVA). Dosages: >65 kg IV a total of 100 mg; 6–10 mg given **IV Bolus** over 1–2 min, 60 mg given over 1st hour, 20 mg given over 2nd hour, 20 mg given over 3rd hour, 1.25 mg/kg given over 3 hr for patients <65 kg.

amiodarone, **Cordarone**: Antidysrhythmic. Uses: Severe VT, SVT, atrial fibrillation, VF not controlled by first line agents, cardiac arrest. Dosages: **PO** loading dose 800–1600 mg/day for 1–3 weeks; then 600–800 mg/day for 1 month; maintenance 400 mg/day; **IV** loading dose (first rapid) 150 mg over the first 10 min, then slow 360 mg over the next 6 hours; maintenance 540 mg given over the remaining 18 hours, decrease rate of the slow infusion to 0.5 mg/min.

argatroban, **Argatroban**: Anticoagulant. Uses: Thrombosis, prophylaxis or treatment; percutaneous coronary intervention (PCI), anticoagulation prevention/treatment of thrombosis in heparin-induced thrombocytopenia. Dosages: *Heparin-induced thrombocytopenia/thrombosis syndrome (HIT or HITTS)—IV:* 2 mcg/kg/min (1 mg/mL) give at 6 mL/hr for 50 kg, at 8 mL/hr for 70 kg, at 11 mL/hr for 90 kg, at 13 mL/hr for 110 kg, at 16 mL/hr for 130 kg. *Hepatic dose—continue infusion* 0.5 mcg/kg/min, adjust rate based on aPTT. *PCI in HIT* IV infusion 25 mcg/kg/min and a bolus of 350 mcg/kg given over 3–5 min, check ACT 5–10 min after bolus is completed; proceed if ACT >300 sec.

atracurium, **Tracrium**: Neuromuscular blocker. Uses: Facilitation of tracheal intubation, skeletal muscle relaxation during mechanical ventilation, surgery, or general anesthesia. Dosages: **IV Bolus** 0.3–0.5 mg/kg, then 0.8–0.10 mg/kg 20–45 min after first dose if needed for prolonged procedures.

Atropine: Antidysrhythmic, anticholinergic, antimuscarinic. Parasympatholytic Uses: Bradycardia, 40–50 bpm, bradydysrhythmia, reversal of anticholinesterase agents, insecticide poisoning, blocking cardiac vagal reflexes, decreasing secretions before surgery, antispasmodic with GU, biliary surgery, bronchodilator. Dosages: ***bradycardia/bradydysrhythmias* IV bolus** 0.5–1 mg given every 3–5 min, not to exceed 2 mg. ***Organophosphate poisoning* IM/IV** 2 mg every hour until muscarinic symptoms disappear, may need 6 mg every hour. ***Presurgery* SC/IM/IV** 0.4–0.6 mg before anesthesia.

cosyntropin, **Cortrosyn:** Pituitary hormone. Uses: Testing adrenalcortical function. Dosage: **IM/IV** 0.25–1 mg between blood sampling.

dexmedetomidine, **Precedex:** Sedative, alpha-2 adrenoceptor agonist. Uses: Sedation in mechanically ventilated, intubated patients ICU. Dosages: **IV** loading dose of 1 mcg/kg over 10 min then 0.2–0.7 mcg/kg/hr, do not use for more than 24 hr.

diltiazem, **Cardizem:** Uses: Calcium channel blocker. **IV:** Atrial fibrillation, flutter, paroxysmal supraventricular tachycardia. Dosages: **IV Bolus** 0.25 mg/kg over 2 min initially, then 0.35 mg/kg may be given after 15 min; if no response, may give **Continuous Infusion** 5–15 mg/hr for up to 24 hr.

dobutamine, **Dobutrex:** Adrenergic direct-acting Beta 1-agonist, cardiac stimulant. Uses: Cardiac decompensation due to organic heart disease or cardiac surgery. Dosages: **IV infusion** 2.5–10 mcg/kg/min; may increase to 40 mcg/kg/min if needed.

dopamine, **Intropin:** Adrenergic. Uses: Shock, increased perfusion, hypotension. Dosages: ***Shock* IV infusion** 2–5 mcg/kg/min, not to exceed 50 mcg/kg/min, titrate to patient's response.

drotrecogin alfa, **Xigris:** Thrombolytic agent. Uses: Severe sepsis associated with organ dysfunction. Dosages: **IV infusion** 24 mcg/kg/hr over 96 hr.

epinephrine: Bronchodilator nonselective adrenergic agonist, vasopressor. Uses: Acute asthmatic attacks, hemostasis, bronchospasm, anaphylaxis, allergic reactions, cardiac arrest, adjunction in anesthesia, shock. Dosages: ***Asthma* Inhaler** 1–2 puffs of 1:100 or 2.25% racemic every 15 min. ***Bronchodilator* SC/IM** 0.1–0.5 mg (1:1000 sol) every 10–15 min–4 hr, max 1 mg/dose. ***Anaphylactic reaction/asthma* SC/IM** 0.1–0.5 mg, repeat every 10–15 min, max 1 mg/dose; epinephrine suspension 0.5 mg **SC,** may repeat 0.5–1.5 mg every 6 hr. ***Cardiac arrest* (ACLS) IV** 1 mg every 3–5 min; **Endotracheal** 2–2.5 mg **IC** 0.3–0.5 mg.

eptifibatide, **Integrilin:** Antiplatelet agent. Uses: Acute coronary syndrome including those undergoing PCI. Dosages: ***Acute coronary*** *syndrome* **IV Bolus** 180 mcg/kg as soon as diagnosed, then **IV Contuous** 2 mcg/kg/min until discharge or CABG up to 72 hr. *PCI in patient's without acute coronary syndrome* **IV Bolus** 180 mcg/kg given immediately before PCI; then 2 mcg/kg/min for 18 hr and a second 180 mcg/kg bolus, 10 min after 1st bolus; continue infusion for up to 18–24 hr.

esmolol, **Brevibloc:** Beta-adrenergic blocker (antidysrhythmic II). Uses: Supraventricular tachycardia, noncompensatory sinus tachycardia, hypertensive crisis, intraoperative and postoperative tachycardia and hypertension. Dosages: **IV** loading dose 500 mcg/kg/min over 1 min; maintenance 50 mcg/kg/min for 4 min; if no response in 5 min, give second loading dose; then increase infusion to 100 mcg/kg/min for 4 min; if no response, repeat loading dose, then increase maintenance infusion by 50 mcg/kg/min (max of 200 mcg/kg/min), titrate to patient response.

etomidate, **Amidate:** General anesthetic. Induction of general anesthesia. Dosages: **IV** 0.2–0.6 mg/kg over 1/2–1 min.

fenoldopam, **Corlopam:** Antihypertensive, vasodilator. Uses: Hypertensive crisis, malignant hypertension. Dosages: **IV** 0.01–1.6 mcg/kg/min.

fentanyl, **Fentanyl:** Opiod analgesic. Uses: Preoperatively, postoperatively; adjunct to general anesthetic, adjunct to regional anesthesia; Fentanyl Oralet: Anesthesia as premedication, conscious sedation. Dosages: *Anesthetic* **IV** 25–100 mcg (0.7–2 mcg/kg) every 2–3 min prn. *Anesthesia supplement* **IV** 2–20 mcg/kg; **IV Infusion** 0.025–0.25 mcg/kg/min. *Induction and maintenance* **IV Bolus** 5–40 mcg/kg. *Preoperatively* **IM** 0.05–0.1 mg every 30–60 min before surgery. *Postoperatively* **IM** 0.05–0.1 mg every 1–2 hr prn.

hetastarch, **Hespan:** Plasma expander. Uses: Plasma volume expander, hypovolemia. Dosages: **IV Infusion** 500–1000 mL (30–60 g), total dose dose not to exceed 1500 mL/day, not to exceed 20 mL/kg/hr (hemorrhagic shock).

isoproterenol, **Isuprel:** Beta-adrenergic agonist. Uses: Bronchospasm, asthma, heart block, ventricular Dysrhythmias, shock. Dosages: *Asthma, Bronchospasms* **SL** 10–20 mg every 6–8 hr, max 60 mg/day; **INH** 1 puff, may repeat in 2–5 min, maintenance 1–2 puffs 4–6 times/day; **IV** 10–20 mcg during anesthesia. *Shock* **IV Infusion** 0.5–5 mcg/min. 1 mg/500 mL D5W, titrate to BP, CVP, hourly urine output.

labetalol, **Normodyne**: Antihypertensive, antianginal. Uses: Mild to moderate hypertension; treatment of severe hypertension. Dosages: **Hypertension** PO 100 mg bid; may be given with a diuretic; may increase to 200 mg bid after 2 days; may continue to increase every 1–3 days; maximum 2400 mg/day in divided doses. **Hypertensive Crisis IV Infusion** 200 mg/160 mL D5W, infuse at 2 mL/min; stop infusion at desired response, repeat every 6–8 hr as needed; **IV Bolus** 20 mg over 2 min, may repeat 40–80 mg every 10 min, not to exceed 300 mg.

Lidocaine: Antidysrhythmic (Class Ib). Uses: Ventricular tachycardia, ventricular Dysrhythmias during cardiac surgery, MI, digitalis toxicity, cardiac catheterization. Dosages: **IV Bolus** 50–100 mg (1 mg/kg) over 2–3 min, repeat every 3–5 min, not to exceed 300 mg in 1 hr; begin **IV Infusion; IV infusion** 20–50 mcg/kg/min; IM 200–300 mg (4.3 mg/kg) in deltoid muscle, may repeat in 1–1½ hr if needed.

midazolam, **Versed**: Sedative, hypnotic, antianxiety. Uses: Preoperative sedation, general anesthesia induction, sedation for diagnostic endoscopic procedures, intubation. Dosages: **Preoperative sedation** IM 0.07–0.08 mg/kg ½–1 hr before general anesthesia. **Induction of general anesthesia** IV (unpremedicated patients) 0.3–0.35 mg/kg over 30 sec, wait 2 min, follow with 25% of initial dose if needed; (premedicated patients) 0.15–0.35 mg/kg over 20–30 sec, allow 2 min for effect. **Continuous infusion for intubation (critical care)** IV 0.01–0.05 mg/kg over several min; repeat at 10–15 min intervals, until adequate sedation; then 0.02–0.10 mg/kg/hr by continuous infusion; adjust as needed.

milrinone, **Primacor**: Inotropic/vasodilator agent with phosphodiesterase activity. Uses: Short-term management of advanced CHF that has not responded to other medication; can be used with digitalis. Dosages: **IV bolus** 50 mcg/kg given over 10 min; start infusion of 0.375–0.75 mcg/kg/min; reduce dose in renal impairment.

naloxone, **Narcan**: opiod-agonist, antidote. Uses: Respiratory depression induced by opiods, pentazocine, propoxyphene; refractory circulatory shock, asphyxia neonatorum, coma, hypotension. Dosages: **Opiod-induced respiratory depression** IV/SC/IM 0.4–2 mg; repeat every 2–3 min if needed. **Postoperative opiod-induced respiratory depression** IV 0.1–0.2 mg every 2–3 min prn. **Opiod overdose** IV/SC/IM 0.4 mg (10 mcg/kg) (not opioid dependant) may repeat every 2–3 min (opiod dependant).

nesiritide, **Natrecor:** Vasodilator. Uses: Acutely decompensated CHF. Dosages: **IV Bolus** 2 mcg/kg, then **IV Infusion** 0.01 mcg/kg/min nitroglycerine: Coronary vasodilator, antianginal. Uses: chronic stable angina pectoris prophylaxis of angina pain, CHF associated with AMI, controlled hypotension in surgical procedures. Dosages: SL, transdermal, topical doses available. IV infusion uses listed only **IV** 5 mcg/min, then increase by 5 mcg/min every 3–5 min; if no response after 20 mcg/min, increase by 10–20 mcg/min until desired response.

nitroprusside, **Nitropress:** Antihypertensive, vasodilator. Uses: Hypertensive crisis, to decrease bleeding by creating hypotension during surgery, acute heart failure. Dosages: **IV infusion** dissolve 50 mg in 2–3 mL of D5W, then dilute in 250–1000 mL of D5W; infuse at 0.5–8 mcg/min.

norepinephrine, **Levophed:** Adrenergic. Uses: Acute hypotension, shock. Dosages: **IV Infusion** 8–12 mcg/min titrated to BP.

pancuronium, **Pavulon:** Neuromuscular blockade. Uses: Facilitation of endotracheal intubation, skeletal muscle relaxation during mechanical intubation, surgery or general anesthesia. Dosages: **IV** 0.04–0.1 mg/kg, then 0.01 mg/kg every ½–1hr.

phenylephrine, **Neo-Synephrine:** adrenergic, direct acting. Uses: Hypotension, paroxysmal supraventricular tachycardia, shock, maintain BP for spinal anesthesia. Dosages: *Hypotension* SC/IM 2–5 mg, may repeat every 10–15 min if needed, do not exceed initial dose; **IV** 50–100 mcg, may repeat every 10–15 min if needed, do not exceed initial dose. *SVT* IV Bolus 0.5–1 mg given rapidly, not to exceed prior dose by >0.1 mg, total dose ≤1 mg. *Shock* IV Infusion 10 mg/500 mL D5W given 100–180 mcg/min, then maintenance of 40–60 mcg/min.

procainamide, **Pronestyl:** Antidysrhythmic. Uses: Life-threatening ventricular dysrhythmias. Dosages: *Atrial Fibrillation/PAT* PO 1–1.25 g; may give another 750 mg if needed; if no response, 500 mg–1 g every 2 hr until desired response; maintenance 50 mg/kg in divided doses every 6 hr. *Ventricular Tachycardia* PO 1g; maintenance 50 mg/kg/day given in 3-hour intervals; **SUS Release** 500 mg–1.25 g every 6 hr. *Other Dysrhythmias* IV Bolus 100 mg every 5 min, given 25–50 mg/min, not to exceed 500 mg; or 17 mg/kg total, then **IV Infusion** 2–6 mg/min.

propofol, **Diprivan:** General anesthetic. Uses: Induction or maintenance of anesthesia as part of balanced anesthetic technique; sedation in mechanically ventilated patients. Dosages: ***Induction IV*** 2–2.5 mg/kg, approximately 40 mg every 10 sec until induction onset. ***Maintenance IV*** 0.1–0.2 mg/kg/min (6–12 mg/kg/hr). ***ICU sedation IV*** 5 mcg/kg/min over 5 min; may give 5–10 mcg/kg/min over 5–10 min until desired response.

rocuronium, **Zemuron:** Neuromuscular blocker (nondepolarizing). Uses: Facilitation of endotracheal intubation, skeletal muscle relaxation during mechanical ventilation, surgery or general anesthesia. Dosages: ***Intubation IV*** 0.6 mg/kg.

streptokinase, **Streptase:** Thrombolytic enzyme. Uses: Deep vein thrombosis, pulmonary embolism, arterial thrombosis, arteriovenous cannula occlusion, lysis of coronary artery thrombi after MI, acute evolving transmural MI. Dosages: ***Lysis of coronary artery thrombi IC*** 20,000 units, then 2,000 international units/min over 1 hour as ***IV Infusion***. ***Arteriovenous cannula occlusion IV Infusion*** 250,000 international units/2 mL solution into occluded limb of cannula run over ½ hour; clamp for 2 hours, aspirate contents; flush with NaCl solution and reconnect. ***Thrombosis/embolism/DVT/pulmonary embolism IV Infusion*** 250,000 international units over ½ hour, then 100,000 international units/hr for 72 hr for deep vein thrombosis; 100,000 international units/hr over 24–72 hr for pulmonary embolism; 100,000 international units/hr for 24–72 hr for arterial thrombosis or embolism. ***Acute evolving transmural MI IV Infusion*** 1,500,000 international units diluted to a volume of 45 mL; give within 1 hr; intracoronary **Infusion** 20,000 international units by **Bolus,** then 2,000 international units/min for 1 hr, total dose 140,000 international units.

succinylcholine, **Anectine:** Neuromuscular blocker (depolarizing—ultra short). Uses: Facilitation of endotracheal intubation, skeletal muscle relaxation during orthopedic manipulations. Dosages: **IV** 0.6 mg/kg, then 2.5 mg/min as needed; **IM** 2.5 mg/kg, not to exceed 150 mg.

tenecteplase, **TNKase:** Thrombolytic enzyme. Uses: acute myocardial infarction. Dosages: *Adults <60 kg:* **IV Bolus** 30 mg, give over 5 sec. *Adult <70 kg:* **IV Bolus** 35 mg, give over 5 sec, *Adult ≥70–<80 kg:* **IV Bolus** 40 mg, give over 5 sec, *Adult ≥80–<90 kg:* **IV Bolus** 45 mg, over 5 sec, *Adult ≥90 kg:* **IV Bolus** 50 mg, give over 5 sec.

tirofiban, **Aggrastat:** Antiplatelet. Uses: Acute coronary syndrome in combination with heparin. Dosages: **IV** 0.4 mcg/kg/min x 30 min, then 0.1 mcg/kg/min for 12–24 hr after angioplasty or atherectomy.

tubocurarine, **Tubarine:** Neuromuscular blockade. Uses: Facilitation of endotracheal intubation, skeletal muscle relaxation during mechanical ventilation, surgery or general anesthesia. Dosages: **IV Bolus** 0.4–0.5 mg/kg, then 0.8–0.10 mg/kg 20–45 min after 1st dose if needed for long procedures.

urokinase, **Abbokinase:** Thrombolytic enzyme. Uses: Venous thrombosis, pulmonary embolism, arterial thrombosis, arterial embolism, arterio-venous cannula occlusion, lysis of coronary artery thrombi after MI. Dosages: *Lysis of pulmonary emboli* IV 4,400 international units/kg/hr for 12–24 hr, not to exceed 200 mL; then **IV** heparin, then anticoagulants. *Coronary artery thrombosis* **Instill** 6,000 international units/min into occluded artery for 1–2 hr after giving **IV Bolus** of heparin 2,500–10,000 units. May also give as **IV Infusion** 2 million–3 million units over 45–90 min. *Venous catheter occlusion* **Instill** 5,000 international units into line, wait 5 min, then aspirate, repeat aspiration attempts every 5 min for $^1/_2$ hr; if occlusion has not been removed, cap line and wait $^1/_2$–1 hr, then aspirate; may need 2nd dose if still occluded.

vasopressin, **Pitressin:** Pituitary hormone, vasoconstrictor. Uses: Diabetes insipidus (nonnephrogenic/nonpsychogenic), abdominal distention postoperatively, bleeding esophageal varices, sepsis. Dosages: *Diabetes insipidus* IM/SC 5–10 units twice a day–four times a day as needed; **IM/SC** 2.5–10 units every 2–3 days for chronic therapy. *Abdominal distention* IM 5 units, then every 3–4 hr, increasing to 10 units if needed. *Sepsis* **IV Infusion** 0.03 units/hr, may titrate up to 0.04 units/hr for BP.

Symbols and Abbreviations

↑	increase
↑↑	greatly increased
↓	decrease
↓↓	greatly decreased
→	leads to, causes
<	less than
≥	less than or equal to
>	greater than
≥	greater than or equal to
/	per, or, divided by
%	percent
(–)	negative
(+)	positive
°	degrees
μ	micro
AAA	abdominal aortic aneurysm
AAD	antibiotic-associated diarrhea
Ab	antibodies
ABG	arterial blood gas
AChr	acetylcholine receptor
ACS	acute coronary syndrome
ACTH	adrenocorticotropic hormone
ACV	assist controlled ventilation
ADH	antidiuretic hormone
$AgNO_3$	silver nitrate aqueous solution
AIS	acute ischemic stroke
A-line	arterial line
AMI	acute myocardial infarction
aPTT	activated partial thromboplastin time
ARDS	adult respiratory distress syndrome
AV	atrial-ventricular
BCP	birth control pills
BE	base excess
BiPAP	bilevel positive airway pressure
BM	bowel movement
BMI	body mass index
BNP	B-type natriuretic peptide
BP	blood pressure
bpm	breaths or beats per minute
BSA	body surface area
BSI	bispectral index monitoring
BUN	blood urea nitrogen
C	Celsius or cervical spine
CAD	coronary artery disease
CAM-ICU	Confusion Assessment Method for the Intensive Care Unit
CAP	community acquired pneumonia
CAPP	coronary artery perfusion pressure
CASS	continuous aspiration of subglottic secretions

Symbols and Abbreviations—*Cont'd*

CAVH .. continuous arteriovenous hemofiltration

CBC . . . . complete blood count

C&DB . . . . cough and deep breathe

CDC . . . . Centers for Disease Control

CEMRI . . . . contrast enhanced magnetic resonance imaging

CHF . . . . . congestive heart failure

CHO . . . . carbohydrates

CI . . . . cardiac index

CK . . . . creatine kinase

CK MB . . . . creatine kinase myocardial band

CLRT . . . . continuous lateral rotation therapy

cm . . . . centimeters

CMP . . . . complete metabolic panel

CMV . . . . . controlled mechanical ventilation

CNS . . . . central nervous system

CO . . . . . . cardiac output, carbon monoxide

CO_2 . . . . carbon dioxide

COHgb . . . . . . carboxyhemoglobin

COPD . . . . chronic obstructive pulmonary disease

CPAP . . . . continuous positive airway pressure

CPIS . . . . clinical pulmonary infection score

CPOT . . . . Critical Care Pain Observation Tool

CPP . . . . cerebral perfusion pressure

CPR . . . . cardio-pulmonary resuscitation

CSF . . . . cerebral spinal fluid

CT . . . . computerized tomography

CVA . . . cerebral vascular accident

CVP . . . . . central venous pressure

CXR . . . . chest x-ray

DBP . . . . . diastolic blood pressure

DI . . . . diabetes insipidus

DIC . . . disseminated intravascular clotting

DKA . . . . . . diabetic ketoacidosis

dL . . . . deciliter

DNI . . . . do not intubate

DNR . . . . do not resuscitate

Do_2 . . . . oxygen delivery

DTR . . . . . . deep tendon reflexes

DVT . . . . . . deep vein thrombosis

D/W . . . . dextrose in water

EBCT . . . . electron beam computed tomography

ECG . . . . electrocardiogram

ECMO . . . . extracorporeal membrane oxygenator

ED . . . . . . emergency department

EEG . . . . . . electroencephalogram

e.g. . . . . for example

Continued

TOOLS

Symbols and Abbreviations—*Cont'd*

ESR . . . erythrocyte sedimentation rate
$ETCO_2$ . . . . end-tidal carbon dioxide
ETOH . . . . alcohol
ETT . . . . endotracheal tube
F . . . . Fahrenheit
FIO_2 . . . . fraction of inspired oxygen
E jFx or EF . . . . . . ejection fraction
FRC . . . . functional residual capacity
GCS . . . . . . Glasgow Coma Scale
GI . . . . gastrointestinal
Gms . . . . grams
GU . . . . genitourinary
HCO_3 . . . . bicarbonate ion
Hct . . . . hematocrit
HCTZ . . . hydrochlorothiazide
HF . . . . heart failure
HFJV . . . high frequency jet ventilation
Hgb . . . . hemoglobin
H_2O . . . . water
HOB . . . . head of bed
HR . . . . heart rate
hr . . . . hour(s)
HRT . . . . . . hormone replacement therapy
HTN . . . . hypertension
Hx . . . . history
IAA . . . . intra-arterial angiography
IABP . . . intra-aortic balloon pump
ICD . . . . implantable cardioverter defibrillator

ICP . . . . intracranial pressure
ICU . . . . intensive care unit
IMV . . . . . intermittent mandatory ventilation
INR . . . . . international normalized ratio
IO . . . . intraosseous
IPP . . . . inspiratory plateau pressure
IRV . . . . . . inverse ratio ventilation
IV . . . . intravenous
IVIG . . . . intravenous immune globulin
J . . . . joules
JVD . . . . jugular venous distention
K^+ . . . . potassium
kg . . . . kilogram
L . . . . liter or lumbar spine
LAP . . . . left atrial pressure
LOC . . . . . . level of consciousness
LPGD . . . . low-profile gastrostomy device
LR . . . . . lactated Ringer's solution
LV . . . . left ventricle
LVEDP . . . . left ventricular end-diastolic pressure
LVF . . . . left ventricular failure
LVSWI . . . . . left ventricular stroke work index
m . . . . meter
MAP . . . . . . mean arterial pressure

Continued

Symbols and Abbreviations—*Cont'd*

mcg . . . . microgram
mEq . . . . milliequivalent
mg . . . . milligram
MI . . . . myocardial infarction
min . . . . minute
mL . . . . milliliter
mm . . . . millimeter
mm Hg . . . . millimeters of
mercury
mmol . . . . millimole
MODS . . . . multiple organ
dysfunction
syndrome
MRA . . . . magnetic resonance
angiography
MRI . . . . magnetic resonance
imaging
MRSA . . . . . . methicillin-resistant
*staphylococcus
aureus*
MS . . . . musculoskeletal
MVC . . . . motor vehicle crash
Na^+ . . . . sodium
NaCl . . . . sodium chloride
$NaHCO_3$ . . . . . sodium bicarbonate
NCV . . . . nerve conduction
velocity
NDT . . . . nasoduodenal tube
NGT . . . . nasogastric tube
NJT . . . . nasojejunal tube
nmol . . . . nanomole
NPO . . . . nothing by mouth
NTG . . . . nitroglycerin
N/V . . . . nausea/vomiting

O_2 . . . . oxygen
OD . . . . overdose
PAC . . . . premature atrial
contraction
$PaCO_2$ . . . . partial pressure of
carbon dioxide in
arterial blood
PAD . . . . pulmonary artery
diastolic pressure
PAH . . . . pulmonary arterial
hypertension
PaO_2 . . . . partial pressure of
oxygen in arterial
blood
P_AO_2 . . . . partial pressure of
alveolar oxygen
PAP . . . . pulmonary artery
pressure
PAP_m . . . . mean pulmonary
artery pressure
PAS . . . . pulmonary artery
systolic pressure
PASG . . . . . pneumatic antishock
garment
$PbtO_2$ . . . . partial pressure of
brain tissue
oxygen
PCI . . . . . percutaneous coronary
intervention
PCO_2 . . . . partial pressure of
carbon dioxide
PCWP . . . . . . pulmonary capillary
wedge pressure
PEA . . . . pulseless electrical
activity

Continued

TOOLS

Symbols and Abbreviations—*Cont'd*

PEEP . . . . . positive end-expiratory pressure

PEG. . . . percutaneous endoscopic gastrostomy

PEJ . . . . percutaneous endoscopic jejunostomy

PET . . . . positron emission tomography

PFT . . . . pulmonary function tests

P$_{ET}$CO$_2$ . . . . partial pressure of carbon dioxide at the end of expiration

P/F ratio. . . . . PaO$_2$/FIO$_2$

pH . . . . potential of hydrogen

po. . . . . by mouth, orally

PO$_2$ . . . partial pressure of oxygen

PQRST. . . . . . palliative/provoking, quality, radiation, severity, timing

prn . . . . as needed

PSV . . . . pressure support ventilation

PT/PTT . . . . prothrombin time/ partial thrombo- plastin time

PVC . . . . premature ventricular contraction

PVR. . . . . pulmonary vascular resistance

PVRI . . . . pulmonary vascular resistance index

RA . . . . right atrium

RAP. . . . . right atrial pressure

RASS . . . . Richmond Agitation Sedation Scale

REM . . . . rapid eye movement

RBBB . . . . right bundle branch block

RR . . . . respiratory rate

RSWI . . . . . right ventricular stroke work index

rtPA . . . . recombinant tissue plasminogen acti- vator

RV. . . . . right ventricle

RVF . . . . . . right ventricular failure

SAH. . . subarachnoid hemorrhage

SaO$_2$ . . . . oxygen saturation

SAS . . . . Sedation Agitation Scale

SBP. . . . . . systolic blood pressure

SCI . . . . spinal cord injury

ScvO$_2$ . . . . central venous oxygen saturation

sec(s) . . . . second(s)

SGOT. . . . . serum glutamic oxaloacetic transaminase

SGPT . . . . serum glutamic pyruvic transaminase

SI. . . . . stroke index

SIADH. . . . . syndrome of inap- propriate anti- diuretic hormone

SIMV . . . synchronous intermittent mandatory ventilation

SIRS . . . . . systemic inflammatory response syndrome

Continued

214

Symbols and Abbreviations—*Cont'd*

SjvO$_2$	cerebral or jugular venous oxygen saturation	Temp	temperature
SL	sublingual	TIA	transient ischemic attack
SNS	sympathetic nervous system	TnI	troponin I
		TPA	tissue plasminogen activator
SOB	shortness of breath	TPN	total parenteral nutrition
SpO$_2$	saturation of peripheral oxygen via pulse oximetry	TSH	thyroid-stimulating hormone
Stat	immediately	UA	urinalysis
SV	stroke volume	UTI	urinary tract infection
SvO$_2$	systemic venous oxygen saturation	VAC	vacuum-assisted closure
		VAP	ventilator-associated pneumonia
SVR	systemic vascular resistance	VAS	Visual Analog Scale
		VF	ventricular fibrillation
SVT	supraventricular tachycardia	VO$_2$	oxygen consumption
		vol	volume
T	thoracic spine	V/Q	ventilation:perfusion
TBI	traumatic brain injury	VS	vital signs
TBSA	total body surface area	VT	ventricular tachycardia
TEE	transesophageal echocardiogram	V–V	venous-venous
		WBC	white blood cell count

Troubleshooting ECG Problems

- Place leads in the correct position. Incorrect placement can give false readings.
- Avoid placing leads over bony areas.
- In patients with large breasts, place the electrodes under the breast. Accurate tracings are obtained through the least amount of fat tissue.
- Apply tincture of benzoin to the electrode sites if the patient is diaphoretic. The electrodes will adhere to the skin better.

TOOLS

- Shave hair at the electrode site if it interferes with contact between the electrode and skin.
- Discard old electrodes and use new ones if the gel on the back of the electrode dries.

Cable Connections

It is important to know if you are using an American or European cable for ECG monitoring. The colors of the wires differ as shown below.

Monitoring Cable Connections		
USA	Connect To	Europe
White	Right arm	Red
Black	Left arm	Yellow
Red	Left leg	Green
Green	Right leg	Black
Brown	Chest	White

Patient Cable

Monitoring cables contain varying numbers of wires.

- **3- and 4-wire cables:** Allow a choice of limb and augmented leads.
- **5-wire cable:** Allows a choice of limb and augmented leads plus a chest lead.
- **10-wire cable:** Records a 12-lead ECG.

Patient ECG Record

Patient name: _____

Sex   F   M

Heart rate: _____ bpm

• Normal (60–100 bpm)	Y	N
• Bradycardia (<60 bpm)	Y	N
• Tachycardia (>100 bpm)	Y	N

Rhythm

• Regular	Y	N
• Irregular	Y	N
• P waves	Y	N

P Waves (form)

• Normal (upright and uniform)	Y	N
• Inverted	Y	N

P wave associated with QRS   Y   N

PR interval normal (0.12–0.20 sec)   Y   N

P waves and QRS complexes associated with one another   Y   N

QRS Interval

• Normal (0.6–0.10 sec)	Y	N
• Wide (>0.10 sec)	Y	N

Are the QRS complex grouped or not grouped?

Are there any dropped beats?

Is there a compensatory or noncompensatory pause?

QT interval: _____

Interpretation: _____

TOOLS

Frequently Used Phone Numbers

Overhead Code:	99/Blue:
Security:	Emergency ext:
Admitting:	
Blood Bank:	
Burn Unit:	
CICU (CCU):	
Chaplain-Pastor:	
Computer Help (IS, IT):	
CT (Computed Tomography):	
Dietary—Dietician:	
ECG—12 Lead:	
ICU:	
Interpreter Services:	
Laboratory:	
Maintenance—Engineering:	
Med-Surg:	
MRI (Magnetic Resonance Imaging):	
Nutrition—Food Services:	
OT (Occupational Therapy):	
PACU (Recovery):	
Pediatrics:	
Pharmacy (Rx):	
Poison Control:	USA – 1-800-222-1222
PT (Physical Therapy):	
Respiratory (RT):	
Social Services:	
Speech Language Pathology (SLP):	
Supervisor—Manager:	
Surgery—Inpatient (OR):	

Continued

Surgery—Day/Outpatient:	
Telemetry Unit:	
X-ray:	

Community Resources

Abuse/Assault—Physical/Sexual	
■ Children	
■ Women	
■ Rape/Sexual	
■ Men	
■ Elderly	
Abuse—Substance	
■ Alcohol	
■ Drug	
Communicable Disease Programs	
■ AIDS	
■ Hepatitis	
■ TB	
Food/Clothing	
■ Food Kitchen	
■ Meals on Wheels	
■ Salvation Army	
Shelters/Homeless	
Mental Health	
■ Suicide	

Continued

TOOLS

Medical/Hospitals	
■ State Program	
■ Dept. of Health	
■ Free Clinics	
Teen/Children	
■ Immunization	
■ Pregnancy	
■ Runaway	
Other	

Basic English-to-Spanish Translation

English Phrase	Pronunciation	Spanish Phrase
Introductions—Greetings		
Hello	**oh**-lah	Hola
Good morning	**bweh**-nohs **dee**-ahs	Buenos días
Good afternoon	**bweh**-nohs **tahr**-dehs	Buenos tardes
Good evening	**bweh**-nahs **noh**-chehs	Buenas noches
My name is	*meh **yah**-moh*	Me llamo
I am a nurse	soy lah oon en-fehr-**meh**-ra	Soy la enfermera
What is your name?	**koh**-moh seh **yah**-mah oo-**sted?**	¿ Cómo se llama usted?

English Phrase	Pronunciation	Spanish Phrase
How are you?	**koh**-moh eh-**stah** **oo**-**stehd?**	¿Como esta usted?
Very well	*mwee b' yehn*	Muy bien
Thank you	**grah**-s'yahs	Gracias
Yes, No	**see,** noh	Sí, No
Please	pohr fah-**vohr**	Por favor
You're welcome	deh **nah**-dah	De nada
Assessment—Areas of the Body		
Head	kah-**beh**-sah	Cabeza
Eye	**oh**-hoh	Ojo
Ear	oh-**ee**-doh	Oído
Nose	nah-**reez**	Nariz
Throat	gahr-**gahn**-tah	Garganta
Neck	**kweh**-yoh	Cuello
Chest, Heart	**peh**-choh, kah-rah-**sohn**	Pecho, corazón
Back	eh-**spahl**-dah	Espalda
Abdomen	ahb-**doh**-mehn	Abdomen
Stomach	eh-**stoh**-mah-goh	Estómago
Rectum	**rehk**-toh	Recto
Penis	**peh**-neh	Pene
Vagina	vah-**hee**-nah	Vagina
Arm, Hand	**brah**-soh, **mah**-noh	Brazo, Mano
Leg, Foot	p'**yehr**-nah, p'**yeh**	Pierna, Pie
Assessment—History		
Do you have...	T'**yeh**-neh oo-**stehd**...	¿Tiene usted...
■ Difficulty breathing?	di-fi-kul-**thad** par-rehspee-**rahr**	¿Dificultad para respirar?
■ Chest pain?	doh-**lorh** en el **peh**-chow	¿Dolor en el pecho?
■ Abdominal pain?	doh-**lorh** ab-doh-mee-**nahl**	¿Dolor abdominal?
■ Diabetes?	dee-ah-**beh**-tehs	¿Diabetes?
Are you...	ehs-**tah**	¿Esta...

Continued

English Phrase	Pronunciation	Spanish Phrase
■ Dizzy?	mar-eh-**a**-dho(dha)	¿Mareado(a)?
■ Nauseated?	kahn **now**-say-as	¿Con nauseas?
■ Pregnant?	¿ehm-bah-rah-**sah**-dah?	¿Embarazada?
Are you allergic to any medications?	¿ehs ah-**lehr**-hee-koh ah ahl-**goo**-nah meh-dee-**see**-nah?	¿Es alergico a alguna medicina?
Assessment—Pain		
Do you have pain?	**T'yeh**-neh oo-**stehd** doh-**lorh**?	¿Tiene usted dolor?
Where does it hurt?	dohn-deh leh **dweh**-leh?	¿Donde le duele?
Is the pain...	es oon doh-lor...	¿Es un dolor...
■ Dull?	**Leh**-veh	¿Leve?
■ Aching?	kans-**tan**-teh	¿constante?
■ Crushing?	ah-plahs-**than**-teh?	¿Aplastante?
■ Sharp?	ah-**goo**-doh?	¿Agudo?
■ Stabbing?	ah-**poo**-nya-lawn-teh?	¿Apuñalante?
■ Burning?	Ahr-**d'yen**-the?	¿Ardiente?
Does it hurt when I press here?	Leh dweh-**leh** kwahn-doh ah-pree-eh-toh ah-**kee**?	¿Le duele cuando le aprieto aqui?
Does it hurt to breathe deeply?	S'yen-teh oo-**sted** doh-lor **kwahn**-doh reh-spee-rah pro-foon-dah-**men**-teh?	¿Siente usted dolor cuando respira profundamente?
Does it move to another area?	Lh doh-**lor** zeh moo-eh-veh a oh-tra **ah**-ri-ah	¿El dolor se mueve a otra area?
Is the pain better now?	S'**yen** tey al-goo-nah me-horr-**ee**-ah	¿Siente alguna mejoria?

Communication with a Non-Verbal Patient

Pain	1	2	3	4	5	6	7	8	9	10

Yes		No		Thank You	
Cold		Hot		Sick	
Thirsty			Hungry		

Please Bring:	Empty:
■ Blanket	■ Bed Pan
■ Eyeglasses	■ Urinal
■ Dentures	■ Trash
■ Hearing Aids	Raise – Lower:
	■ Head
	■ Legs

Oral Care	Bath		Shower
TV	Lights	On	Off

Web Resources for Evidence-Based Practices in Critical Care

Agency for Healthcare Research & Quality . . . . www.ahrq.gov
Algorithms for the Medical ICU . . . . www.clevelandclinicmeded.com/micu
American Association of Critical-Care Nurses . . . . www.aacn.org
American College of Cardiology . . . . www.acc.org
American Heart Association . . . . www.americanheart.org

TOOLS

American Thoracic Society . . . . www.thoracic.org
Brain Dysfunction in
    Critically Ill Patients . . . . http://www.icudelirium.org/delirium/
Centers for Disease Control & Prevention . . . . www.cdc.gov
Emergency Nurses Association . . . . www.ena.org
Healthcare Freeware (2005) . . . . . . www.healthcarefreeware.com/icu.htm
Institute for Healthcare Improvement
    Critical Care. . . . . www.ihi.org/IHI/Topics/CriticalCare/
Internet Stroke Center . . . . www.strokecenter.org
Medscape . . . . www.medscape.com
National Guideline Clearinghouse . . . . www.guideline.gov
National Heart Lung & Blood Institute . . . . www.nhlbi.nih.gov
National Spinal Cord Injury Association . . . . www.spinalcord.org
Sedation, Analgesia, and Neuromuscular
    Blockade in the ICU . . . . www.mc.vanderbilt.edu/surgery/
                                   trauma/Protocols/SedationAnal-
                                   gesiaGuidelines.pdf
Surviving Sepsis Campaign . . . . . . www.survivingsepsis.org/implement/
                                   bundles

Selected References

Badesch DB, Abman SH, Simonneau G, Rubin LJ, McLaughlin VV. Medical therapy for pulmonary hypertension. Chest. 2007;131(6):1917–1928.

Broscious SK, Castagnola J. Chronic kidney disease: Acute manifestation and role of critical care nurses. Crit Care Nurs. 2006;26(4):17–27.

Gay SE, Ankney N, Cochran J, Highland KB. Critical care challenges in the adult ECMO patient. Dimens Crit Care Nurs. 2005;24(4):157–162.

Holcomb SS. Diabetes insipidus. Dimens Crit Care Nurs. 2002;21(3):94–97.

Kaplow R, Hardin SR. *Critical Care Nursing: Synergy for Optimal Outcomes.* Boston, MA: Jones and Bartlett; 2007.

Levy MM, Fink MP, Marshall JC, Abraham E, Angus D, et al. 2001 SSCM/ESICM/ACCP/ATS/SIS International Sepsis Definitions Conference. Crit Care Med. 2003;31(4):1250–1256.

Martin CG. Nursing care of the patient undergoing coronary artery bypass grafting. J Cardiovas Nurs. 2006;21(2):109–117.

Metules T. Unstable angina: Is your care up to snuff? RN. 2005;68(2):22–27.

O'Connor KJ, Wood KE, Lord K. Intensive management of organ donors to maximize transplantation. Crit Care Nurs. 2006;26(2):94–100.

Pfadt, E, Carlson DS. Acute adrenal crisis. Nurs. 2006;36(8):80.

Rosenthal LD. Carbon monoxide poisoning. Am J Nurs. 2006;106(3):40–46.

Russ A. *Drug Pocket Clinical Reference Guide*. 5th ed. Hermosa Beach, Ca: Borm Bruckmeier; 2006.

Shaughnessy L. Massive pulmonary embolism. Crit Care Nurs. 2007;27(1): 39–50.

Smeltzer SC, Bare BG. *Brunner & Suddarth's Textbook of Medical-Surgical Nursing*. 10th ed. Philadelphia, PA: LWW; 2004.

Sole ML, Klein DG, Moseley MJ. *Introduction to Critical Care Nursing*. 4th ed. St. Louis, MO: Elsevier Saunders; 2005.

Taylor MM. ARDS diagnosis and management. Dimens Crit Care Nurs. 2005;24(5):197–207.

Taylor MM. ARDS diagnosis and management: Implications for the critical care nurse. Dimens Crit Care Nurs. 2005;24(5):197–207.

Timmerman RA. A mobility protocol for critically ill adults. Dimens Crit Care Nurs. 2007;26(5):175–178.

Warkentin TE, Greinacher A. Heparin-induced thrombocytopenia: Recognition, treatment, and prevention: The seventh ACCP conference on Antithrombotic and thrombolytic therapy. Chest. 2004;126(3): 311s—337s.

Williams C. Fluid resuscitation in burn patients 1: Using formulas. Nurs Times. 2008;104(14):28–29.

Williams WJ. *Williams Hematology*. 7th ed. New York, NY: McGraw-Hill; 2006.

Illustration Credits

Pages 65 and 74 from Jones: ECG Notes, FA Davis, Philadelphia, 2005.

Pages 68, 69, and 75 from Hopkins: Med Surg Notes, FA Davis, Philadelphia, 2007.

Pages 71–74, and 76–80 from Armstrong Medical Industries, Inc. Lincolnshire, IL.

TOOLS

Page 86 adapted from Singh N, Rogers P, Atwood CW, etal: Short-course empiric antibiotic therapy for patients with pulmonary infiltrates in the intensive care unity. American Journal of Respiratory and Critica IC are Medicine, 162: 505-511, 2000 in Beers MH :The Merck manual, 18th edition.

Pages 112 and 198 from Myers: RNotes, 2e, FA Davis, Philadelphia, 2006.

Page: 114 from The Lancet, Vol. 304, Teasdale Gand Jennett B. Assessment of Coma and Impaired Consciousness: A Practical Scale, Page4, Copyright (1994), with permission from Elsevier.